Medicaid and the Limits
of State Health Reform

Medicaid and the Limits of State Health Reform

Michael S. Sparer

TEMPLE UNIVERSITY PRESS
Philadelphia

Temple University Press, Philadelphia 19122
Copyright © 1996 by Temple University
All rights reserved
Published 1996
Printed in the United States of America

⊛ The paper used in this publication meets the requirements of the American
National Standard for Information Sciences — Permanence of Paper for Printed
Library Materials, ANSI Z39.48–1984

Text design by Gary Gore

Library of Congress Cataloging-in-Publication Data

Sparer, Michael S.
    Medicaid and the limits of state health reform / Michael S. Sparer.
        p.   cm.
    Includes bibliographical references and index.
    ISBN 1-56639-433-3 (cloth : alk. paper). — ISBN 1-56639-434-1
(pbk. : alk. paper)
    1. Health care reform — United States — States.   2. Medicaid —
Government policy — United States — States.   I. Title.
RA398.A3S63   1996
362.1′0973 — dc20   95-47190

For Jo

Contents

Acknowledgments

I could not have written this book without the love and support of my wife, Jo. My first and most important debt, in so very many ways, is thus to her. We are a team.

I'm also extremely grateful to Larry Brown, who is the ideal colleague: supportive, insightful, and a good friend. Jim Fossett, Larry Jacobs, Marty Levin, Shep Melnick, Dick Nathan, Deborah Stone, and Frank Thompson all offered useful advice and constant encouragement. Sylvia Law is both a close friend and a valued advisor. Michael Ames, my editor at Temple, had faith that I could turn a dissertation into a book. Along with faith, he provided sound editorial judgment.

I'd also like to thank the dozens of government officials who took time away from their busy schedules and let me interview them. Much of this book is simply their story.

An earlier version of chapter 5 appeared in the journal *Health Affairs* (spring 1993). An earlier version of chapter 8 appears in the *Journal of Health Politics, Policy and Law* (summer 1996).

Carl Rubin, Paul Fishstein, Jim Oppenheim, and George West each provide a special friendship that I rely on and need.

Finally, I'd like to acknowledge how my life, and thus this book, is shaped by my family. The memory of my father, Edward Sparer, inspires and challenges me. My mother, Tanya Sparer, gave me the book "The Little Engine That Could" and convinced me to say "I think I can." My sisters Ellen and Carol, Jo's siblings Donna and Allen, and all the members of their families provide important roots in my family tree. My daughters, Emily and Madeline, spent countless hours upstairs because Daddy was working in his office downstairs. They should know that my favorite moments are when we're all together (upstairs or downstairs). My girls are the joys of my life.

And Jo — to you I dedicate this book.

Medicaid and the Limits
of State Health Reform

1

The State Role in Health Care Reform: Why Do We Care?

Health Care Reformers Turn to the States

It is by now well known that the United States is the only Western industrialized nation without national health insurance. Following the 1992 presidential elections, however, it seemed that this exceptionalism was about to end. Newly elected President Bill Clinton declared health care reform to be a (very) high domestic priority. Pollsters revealed citizen support for reform. Key interest groups (including health care providers, commercial insurance companies, and much of the business community) voiced support for reform as well. Even leading Republicans generally agreed that there was a "health care crisis" that needed to be addressed.

In the fall of 1993, the president unveiled his plan. The federal government would establish a health insurance benefit package that every American would receive. "Health plans" (mainly large health maintenance organizations) would compete to provide the benefit package. Employers would fund most of the cost, but employees would pay some too, and they would have a fiscal incentive to choose a low-cost plan. Newly formed "health alliances" (quasi-governmental agencies established and administered by state governments) would manage the competition, protecting consumers and employers alike. The newly competitive environment would generate savings (and if it didn't, a national health board would ensure savings by imposing caps on the premiums charged by the plans). There would thus be health insurance (and health security) for all and a gradual reduction in the nation's trillion dollar health care bill.

Soon after the proposal was released, however, the momentum for reform disappeared. Interest groups that supported reform in the abstract opposed key elements of the president's plan, especially the requirement that employers provide insurance to their employees and the proposed caps on insurance premiums. Meanwhile, consumers worried that the emphasis on managed care would eliminate freedom of choice and undermine existing doctor-patient relationships. And the new bureaucracies envisioned by the plan (such as the so-called health alliances) fed Republican arguments that the plan was just another big-government proposal generated by big-spending liberal Democrats.

By the summer of 1994, Congress had rejected the Clinton plan, along with a host of alternative proposals. The 1994 midterm elections then produced a Republican Congress (the first since 1946), an apparent repudiation of Clinton's ambitious domestic agenda. Voters distrusted government's ability to solve the health care crisis (and were persuaded by the Republican's platform of lower taxes and less government).

In this changed political environment, the Clinton administration shifted tactics: the new goal is to encourage states to be the source of health policy innovation. This strategy consists primarily of providing a handful of states with greater discretion when implementing Medicaid, the federal-state health insurance program for the poor. States are encouraged to use this authority to expand the program to cover segments of the uninsured. Tennessee, for example, is implementing a program called TennCare, which offers a choice of managed care plans to nearly 1.5 million low-income persons, a third of whom were previously uninsured.[1] Oregon has a similar program.[2]

Other health care reformers, having acknowledged that national health insurance is off the political agenda, also focus now on the states. The goal is to support state programs for the uninsured. The hope is that innovative state programs will become models emulated elsewhere.

State programs for the uninsured can be divided into several categories. First are efforts to encourage or require employers to provide health insurance to their employees. Hawaii, for example, requires most employers to provide health insurance to their employees.[3] Oregon has a similar requirement, though it is not scheduled to go into effect until 1997. Other states, unwilling to impose employer mandates, provide tax credits (or similar subsidies) to small businesses that provide health insurance to low-income employees.

A second strategy is to use state dollars to pay for private insurance. Minnesota, for example, subsidizes private insurance for families with income below 275 percent of poverty and individuals with income below 100 percent of poverty.[4] This program, called MinnesotaCare, is funded by a special tax imposed on health care providers. Washington State has a similar program, called the Basic Health Plan, which provides subsidized insurance to persons with income below 200 percent of poverty.[5] Washington's program is financed primarily by so-called sin taxes (on alcohol and tobacco) and by a tax on hospitals and HMOs.

Third are initiatives which seek to lower the cost of private health insurance. These programs generally focus on small employers, the group with the largest number of uninsured workers. California, for example, has created a health insurance purchasing pool for small employers. The assumption is that if small employers pool their insurance business, their ability to negotiate lower rates increases. Other states permit insurers to offer "bare bones" health insurance policies (by waiving state laws that require every insurance policy to cover services such as drug treatment or mental health coverage). Still other states impose an actual cap on increases in insurance premiums.

Fourth, and finally, a number of states provide subsidies to those health care providers who care for the uninsured. In 1987, for example, state and local governments spent over $18 billion to cover uncompensated care.[6] In addition, a few states impose a special tax (called a surcharge) on all hospital bills, then distribute the funds collected to hospitals that provide uncompensated care. New York has had such a program for over a decade.

To be sure, these various state programs, taken together, have hardly made a dent in the overall number of uninsured. (Indeed, the number of uninsured continues to rise.) Reformers hope, however, that the failure of national health reform will encourage more states to adopt programs for the uninsured. Perhaps Montana or Missouri will adopt their own employer mandate. Or maybe Alabama or Arkansas will implement a program like Washington's Basic Health Plan. This hope, that states will act as policy laboratories, and that other states will replicate programs that work, has led to an alliance between those who have argued for years that health reform should be led by the states and those who would prefer a national solution but believe it unlikely.

Liberal reformers are not alone, however, in pinning their hopes on the states. The new Republican leaders in Congress, joined by several of the nation's governors, also argue that states should be given increased authority to run health and welfare programs. For example, Republican legislation would turn Medicaid into a block grant, under which states would receive a fixed amount of federal Medicaid dollars, but would be able to spend those dollars with very few (if any) federal strings. One goal of the block grant approach is simply to reduce federal expenditures: federal spending would be capped and controlled. Supporters also suggest, however, that a block grant would enable state policymakers to innovate and contain costs in ways now impossible. This increased authority is the main draw for the nation's governors.

There is, as such, a second and even more unlikely alliance, this one between liberal reformers and conservative cost-cutters, both of whom look to the states as a source of innovation and leadership.[7]

Given the mood of the day, Congress is likely to increase state authority over health care policy and put off indefinitely further consideration of national health insurance. Even if Medicaid is not converted to a block grant, for example, state flexibility under the program will surely increase. Federal regulations governing the quality of health care provided by nursing homes may also be eliminated, replaced (if at all) by an assortment of state regulatory regimes. In time, even Medicare, the federally funded and administered program for the aged and disabled, may be replaced by a collection of state-based insurance initiatives.

The policy implications of this "devolution revolution" are unclear.[8] How will states respond to their increased authority (especially if it is accompanied by a reduction in federal dollars)? What are the strengths and the limits of states as policymakers? Who will win and who will lose?

One source of insight is the literature on state health reform activities. What states have done provides clues as to what states might do. Unfortunately, the literature is surprisingly thin. There are, to be sure, several organizations that do a good job of tracking and reporting state health care policy.[9] There are also a handful of articles and books on recent state health reform activity.[10] By and large, however, the more analytic work focuses on the half dozen states that have enacted comprehensive reform; there is hardly anything written about the other 45. Moreover, even the literature describing the reform leaders needs to be revised. The reform leaders are retreating fast. Washington State, for example, recently rescinded a state law that would have required employers to provide employees with health insurance beginning in 1999. Minnesota repealed its goal of universal coverage by 1997, substituting a goal of 96 percent coverage. Florida, Vermont, and Colorado also retreated from their flirtation with comprehensive reform.

The reduced commitment to reform is hardly surprising. State legislators in 1996 are generally less likely to enact insurance expansions than their state or federal counterparts were in 1994. The Republican revolution is firmly entrenched in many statehouses. Washington State illustrates the point. In 1993, the state's Democratic-controlled legislature enacted a comprehensive health insurance program, one that was hailed by reformers around the country as a model to be emulated. The next year, the Republicans took over the statehouse, and by early 1995 they had repealed the most publicized piece of the reform initiative, the employer mandate.

The 1994 elections are not, however, the only reason that states are not likely to enact universal coverage programs. An obvious obstacle is money: finding new dollars for reform is difficult, especially since state policymakers are no more likely than their federal counterparts to seek tax increases. State innovation is also limited by fear of business exodus. States are in an ongoing interstate competition for business, and state officials worry that if they increase the burdens imposed on the private sector (perhaps by requiring employers to provide health insurance to their employees) then at least some employers will move their businesses elsewhere. A third obstacle is the fear of becoming a welfare magnet. State policymakers worry that if they enact universal insurance, and other states do not, then some uninsured persons might migrate in solely to receive the new benefits.

The changing medical marketplace also makes government action less likely. For example, many big businesses are now forming large health insurance purchasing alliances, thereby gaining discounts and savings that were previously unavailable, and thereby reducing even further their incentive to support programs for the uninsured.

Finally, for those few states who elude the interest-group, institutional, and ideological barriers, there are inter-governmental barriers as well, most notably the Employee Retirement Income and Security Act (known as ERISA), which prohibits states from requiring employers to provide health insurance to their employees. It also prohibits states from regulating or taxing those companies that self-insure.[11] Since nearly 70 percent of all employees work for companies that self-insure, ERISA is a powerful barrier to nearly every state reform initiative. Washington State, for example, could not have implemented its now-repealed employer mandate without an ERISA exemption from Congress. Moreover, despite the rhetoric about the need for state experimentation, Congress has so far been unwilling to exempt states from the restrictions of ERISA: business and labor, which both benefit from the law, lobby vigorously against any waiver applications. Even Hawaii, which in 1983 received the nation's only ERISA exemption, has regularly been rebuffed in its effort to amend its waiver.[12]

Given these barriers to reform, it is unlikely that any state will respond to the new era with either comprehensive insurance expansions or innovative cost-containment measures. Instead, most states will tinker with incremental initiatives. Nearly all will cut Medicaid eligibility and encourage (or require) the remaining beneficiaries to enroll in managed care. Many will enact small-group purchasing pools. Some will subsidize private health insurance for a small minority of the uninsured, primarily women and children. Others will encourage individuals to open tax deferred medical savings accounts. Still others will experiment with purchasing pools for state employees. A few will do as little as possible.

It is impossible to predict, of course, which states will do what in a state-dominated health policy environment. Perhaps one or two (or more) will be surprisingly bold. Others might engage in a discouraging "race to the bottom" (an effort to see which can impose the most draconian cost-containment regime). Most might simply muddle ahead, incrementally adjusting and tinkering.

As discussed earlier, the literature on current state health reform activities provides few clues about future state activity; so far, analysts have focused on just a few states (the so-called reform leaders) and most of the programs studied are brand new. There is, however, another source of guidance and insight that is surprisingly untapped: Medicaid, the federal-state health insurance program for the poor that was enacted in 1965, is in place in all fifty states, and is at the heart of the current debate over national health care policy. This book provides such an examination.

Medicaid: Fifty States, Fifty Programs

Medicaid, like many of the newer state reform initiatives now underway, has clearly benefited millions of persons. The thirty-three million Medicaid beneficiaries have a health insurance card that entitles them to a relatively wide array of services. In some states, the Medicaid benefit package compares favorably with that of typical private policies. And while Medicaid beneficiaries often have difficulty finding doctors who will treat them, poor persons with Medicaid still see physicians far more often than do poor uncovered persons.[13]

At the same time, however, Medicaid has also disappointed those who expected (or hoped) that the program would provide poor persons with health care equal to that of the non-poor. Nearly 50 percent of the nation's poor are not even eligible for coverage. Equally troubling, most Medicaid beneficiaries have long encountered a health care system disinclined to care for poor persons, even if the poor person has a Medicaid card. As a result, millions of Medicaid beneficiaries neither have their own physician nor ready access to a private physician's practice. For these clients, particularly those in the nation's urban areas, medical care is received most often in the emergency rooms of large public hospitals.

Medicaid's failings are due to a range of factors, including low provider physician reimbursement rates, unfriendly administrative bureaucracies, and an undeserved reputation as a health care program only for welfare recipients. More generally, however, each of these problems is exacerbated by a complicated (and convoluted) administrative structure, under which state officials have significant discretion in deciding who in their state receives coverage, what medical benefits are provided, and how much health care providers are paid.

Why has the delegation of authority proved troublesome? Because it has produced inappropriate and inequitable variation in state Medicaid programs (even between programs in states with similar socio-economic conditions and a similar commitment to social welfare) and ongoing intergovernmental tension as federal, state, and even local officials each try to shift costs and responsibilities to the other. Moreover, thirty years of state Medicaid programs have produced compelling evidence that states, contrary to American folklore, are not especially good policy laboratories.

Consider, for example, the interstate variation in the nation's Medicaid program. In California, a family of three with a monthly income below $934 can receive coverage, while a similar family in Alabama needs an income below $149 to qualify. Similarly, a three-person family in Vermont needs income below $900 to qualify, while their neighbors in Maine can have no more than $458. Other border states have similar variation.[14] In Pennsylvania, a hospital that treats a Medicaid client receives in reimbursement approximately 79 percent of the cost of care. In New Jersey, however, a similarly situated hospital receives from Medicaid 105 percent of the cost of care.[15] In twenty-eight states, Medicaid pays for chiropractic services; six states cover hospice care; in no two states, however, do clients receive the same medical benefit package.

Most tellingly, overall Medicaid expenditures vary dramatically, even between states that seem similarly situated. In 1993, New Hampshire spent $5,264 per beneficiary compared to $3,171 by Vermont, and Arkansas spent $3,038 compared to $2,372 spent in Mississippi.[16]

Good and Bad Variation

Variation in state health care policy is not necessarily bad. The health care delivery system in New York City should look very different from its counterpart in rural Idaho. Local needs do differ. Medical practice patterns should reflect local needs. The health care industry also varies by state. Some states have a long history of managed care penetration, while others still resist the movement toward managed care. Some states have a large number of non-profit and public hospitals, while others are dominated by large for-profit hospital chains. Some states train a high percentage of the nation's medical residents, while others barely have a medical education system. These differences all produce variation in medical practice, much of which is appropriate and necessary.

At the same time, there is little justification for the interstate variation that exists in Medicaid. First, the variation raises important normative questions. Why should a low-income resident of California receive Medicaid coverage, while an Alabama resident with the same income is uninsured? Why should a beneficiary in New York have a home attendant, while her counterpart in Indiana goes without? Why should a hospital in Pennsylvania receive far lower reimbursement than a similarly situated facility in New Jersey?

The variation raises policy questions as well. For example, the argument that states can and do act as policy laboratories assumes that policy outcomes in one state will be duplicated in others. The interstate variation in Medicaid programs, however, makes it difficult to generalize about specific Medicaid demonstration projects. TennCare, for example, is a pilot program, presumably testing the viability of combining a mandatory managed care initiative with a significant eligibility coverage expansion. The reproducibility of the TennCare experience is clearly undermined, however, by the vast differences between Tennessee's Medicaid program and those found in other states.

The task (and the challenge) is to develop policies that minimize inappropriate interstate variation and maximize useful interstate variation. To do this, however, requires more knowledge about why the interstate variation in Medicaid (and health care policy more generally) is so pronounced. Why do similar states produce dissimilar programs?

This book examines the issue of Medicaid variation through a comparative case study of the Medicaid programs in California and New York. Why a comparative case study? Because explaining Medicaid variation requires delving deeply into the history and politics of different Medicaid programs. Why look at these states? Because they not only have the nation's two largest Medicaid programs (by far), but also because the interstate variation between the two programs presents a policy puzzle: why do two states with similar economies and a similar commitment to social welfare have such different programs?

The answer to this policy puzzle emerges in the case study found in Chapters Four through Eight. In California, state Medicaid officials enjoy significant bureaucratic discretion and can ensure that provider reimbursement is kept quite low. As a result, even though the state has liberal Medicaid eligibility policies and provides a generous medical benefit package, overall expenditures are relatively low. In New York, in contrast, Medicaid bureaucrats operate within a fragmented, decentralized, and interest-group-dominated political system, in which the key players generally have little interest in pursuing a cost-containment agenda. Medicaid expenditures have soared as a result.

Explaining Medicaid Variation:
The Bureaucratic Discretion Variable

A central question of political science is, "Who governs?"[17] Who determines which government programs are enacted, how such programs are implemented, and to whom public power and resources are distributed?

One answer is that public policy is best understood as a response to the demands of the most effective interest groups in society. Under this paradigm, U.S. politics is society-centered and group-dominated. This view is challenged, however, by the hypothesis that policy decisions typically reflect the interests of key "state actors" (mainly politicians and government bureaucrats), and that societal groups have relatively little input. This alternative explanation suggests that U.S. politics is "state-centered."

The society-centered explanation dominates contemporary political science. The leading proponents are the pluralists, who argue 1) that there are a variety of resources useful in shaping policy (such as money, status, skill, and charisma); 2) that these resources, while not distributed equally, are non-cumulative (the rich man is not necessarily the most skilled); and 3) that most interest groups have access to at least some of these resources. Policy thus emerges, incrementally, through negotiation and compromise between interested groups.[18]

One challenge to the pluralists is that there is an upper-class bias in U.S. politics.[19] The wealthy, for example, are disproportionately influential. So too is the business community. Similarly, in health care politics, the provider community and the insurance industry are more influential than the uninsured or the Medicaid beneficiary. But this view too suggests that political decisions reflect the interests of groups: Government is observer and referee, responding to the agenda of others rather than implementing its own will.

According to some, however, this description of policymaking inaccurately minimizes the role played by public officials. Eric Nordlinger, for example, notes that the policy preferences of public officials are often self-generated (shaped by career goals, or organizational loyalty, or professional expertise, or a perception of the public interest). These officials also have the resources to implement their preferences. For these reasons, he finds it "most implausible that the democratic state — the elected and appointed officials who populate this large, weighty, resource-laden, highly prized ensemble of offices — is consistently unwilling or unable to translate its preferences into public policy when they diverge from those held by the politically weightiest societal groups."[20]

Nordlinger readily concedes that public officials are unlikely to act autonomously in the face of ongoing and overwhelming societal opposition (though he insists that such crises are rare). He also concedes that public officials do respond to societal groups: stubborn autonomy is not a good re-election strategy. The argument, however, is that political science has for too long minimized the importance of the state.

The case study provided in this book contributes to the literature on this debate. In California, state Medicaid officials enjoy significant bureaucratic discretion and have successfully implemented their policy preferences. In New York, in contrast, Medicaid bureaucrats operate within an interest-group–dominated political system, and Medicaid policy is generated through a more pluralistic process.

To be sure, policymaking environments are not fixed. The two states are not ironclad examples of pure models. New York State regulators sometimes act autonomously. Interest groups in California sometimes influence Medicaid policy. But while elements of both models are present in both states, the dominant patterns differ. This finding suggests that the answer to the pluralist versus state-centered debate depends, in part, on the policy and the state examined.

The Organization of the Book

To provide context and background, Chapter Two explores why in the early 1990s health reform became such a potent political issue, why nearly every health reform proposal before the 103rd Congress (including President Clinton's) delegated such significant authority to the states, and why these various health reform initiatives failed.

I then turn to the Medicaid program in Chapter Three, discussing in some detail the intergovernmental bickering that dominates the program, the enormous variation in the fifty state Medicaid programs, the literature which seeks to explain that variation, and the need for a comparative case study to supplement that literature. Chapters Four through Eight then present the comparative case study of the Medicaid programs in California and New York: Chapter Four provides an overview, and the next four chapters discuss nursing home policy, home care policy, hospital policy, and managed care policy respectively. Finally, I discuss in Chapter Nine the lessons suggested by the comparative case study and draw some conclusions about intergovernmental relations, health care politics, and the states' role in a reformed health care system.

2

Congress Considers Health Reform

The Federal Role in Health Care: A Brief History

For much of U.S. history, the federal government was only a minor player in the nation's health care system. During the nineteenth century, for example, federal health care legislation was considered not only unwise but at times even unconstitutional. National health insurance wasn't even debated until 1912, when former President Theodore Roosevelt, campaigning then as a member of the Progressive political party, urged its adoption. But Roosevelt's proposal for universal insurance was quickly labeled "un-American" and "socialistic" by doctors, businessmen, and even union officials and was easily defeated. Later initiatives by Franklin Roosevelt[1] and Harry Truman fared no better.[2]

Lacking either federal leadership or federal funding, state and local governments tried for years to provide a medical safety net. In urban areas, for example, several local governments led "sanitary reform movements," which reduced infectious disease by improving sewage and garbage disposal. Many local governments also established public hospitals to care for the poor and public clinics to provide health services to the community at large. And several states developed specialized institutions for the mentally ill and the developmentally disabled. Despite these efforts, the quantity and quality of government health care programs remained sporadic and generally inadequate.

Following World War II, however, the federal government for the first time became involved in shaping the nation's health care system. Much of the activity was generated by the era of American optimism that arrived with the end of the war. There was now a perception that medical research and specialized medical care would in time conquer nearly all forms of disease. This assumption prompted Congress to use the National Institutes of Health to funnel billions of dollars to academic medical researchers. Congress also enacted the Hill-Burton program, which provided federal funds to stimulate hospital construction and modernization.[3] The policy assumption was that all Americans should have access to the increasingly sophisticated medical care rendered in state-of-the-art hospital facilities. Hill-Burton eventually subsidized the construction of nearly four hundred thousand hospital beds (including many in rural communities).

Congress did more, however, than simply underwrite the establishment of a hospital-based specialty care health delivery system (though it certainly did do that). It also enacted an amendment to the Social Security Act in 1950, which, for the first time, provided federal funds to those states willing to pay health care providers to care for welfare recipients. In retrospect, this program was Medicaid's forerunner. Interestingly, the program passed, despite the conservatism of the day, because of support received from both sides of the national health insurance debate. For proponents of a comprehensive insurance plan, the 1950 amendment was an acceptable, if inadequate, first step. At least some poor persons could now receive previously unavailable medical care. Opponents of national health insurance went along also, both because a medical safety net for the poor would undermine arguments for a more comprehensive health insurance program, and because responsibility for the program was delegated to state officials.

A decade later, in 1960, Congress expanded its "welfare medicine"[4] system for the poor, enacting the Kerr-Mills program, which provided federal funds to states willing to pay health care providers to care for the indigent aged. Two years later, Kerr-Mills was expanded to cover the indigent disabled. These bipartisan initiatives once again deflected support from a Democratic proposal to provide federally funded universal hospital insurance to all of the aged, regardless of income. Instead, participating states would set income eligibility criteria and would share with the federal government all program costs. The result was significant interstate variation: by 1963, five states (California, Massachusetts, Michigan, New York, and Pennsylvania) received approximately 90 percent of the federal Kerr-Mills funds even though they had only 32 percent of the nation's over-sixty-five population.[5]

By delegating responsibility for "welfare medicine" to the states, Congress was continuing the long-standing tradition that welfare programs should be administered and controlled by local officials. U.S. policymakers were long influenced, for example, by the English poor laws (or the early English welfare programs), which limited welfare benefits to the so-called deserving poor (or those persons outside the labor market through no fault of their own), and which required that welfare programs be established, financed, and administered by local governments. Indeed, the power of this tradition, and the influence of a handful of southern congressmen who fought to preserve it, shaped the welfare programs that emerged during the New Deal: the federal government finances and administers the so-called social insurance programs (like Social Security), which most Americans believe are earned rights and not welfare, but the states administer, set policy for, and help finance most so-called welfare programs (such as Aid to Families With Dependent Children), which most Americans believe represent "charity" that should go only to the "deserving poor."

The bifurcated nature of the U.S. medical safety net remained firmly in place in 1965, when Congress, following Lyndon B. Johnson's landslide election, finally enacted two major programs of government-funded health insurance, Medicare and Medicaid. Medicare, which provides a fixed set of health insurance benefits to nearly all of the nation's aged, is considered a "social insurance" program, providing an earned set of benefits. It is financed and administered by the federal government.[6] Medicaid, in contrast, is considered a "welfare" program, providing benefits primarily to the "deserving poor." It is funded jointly by the federal and state governments, and it delegates to state officials significant discretion in determining which poor persons are covered, what benefits are provided, and how much providers are paid.

Interestingly, however, one of the few Medicaid policy areas in which the federal government actually limited state discretion concerned hospital reimbursement. Here the other long-standing federal policy trend reigned supreme: protect and nurture the growing hospital industry. As a result, both Medicaid and Medicare (much like private insurance companies)[7] generally paid any and all hospital bills along with the bills submitted by the specialists who worked in the hospitals.

There was a price to be paid for the blank check given to the hospital industry. First, rising hospital costs helped to drive the nation's health care bill rapidly higher. After all, 44 percent of personal health care expenditures are for hospital services,[8] and between 1970 and 1980 spending on hospital services increased nearly 14 percent annually.[9] Second, the federal government's (rather minimal) efforts to encourage community-based primary care clinics never lived up to expectations. Consider, for example, the neighborhood health center program (now called the community health clinic program) established at the same time as Medicaid and Medicare in 1965. This program provides federal funds to support community-run clinics in poverty stricken areas. The policy assumption is that these clinics can effectively provide coordinated and comprehensive care to otherwise underserved poor persons. The evidence supports the assumption.

The success of the community health center model has not, however, persuaded federal officials to give the program a high priority. As long ago as 1967, for example, federal officials projected that by 1973 there would be more than a thousand clinics,

serving twenty-five million poor persons and receiving direct federal subsidies of more than $3 billion annually.[10] As of 1994, there
are only 627 centers, serving only seven million persons and receiving less than $700 million in direct federal subsidies.[11] The less
than expected financial support was due, in large part, to the rising
costs of the nation's acute care system. Congress was (and is)
spending so much supporting hospital-based care that little was
left over for alternative models.

The first president seriously to challenge the nation's rising hospital bill was Jimmy Carter. In 1977, shortly after his election,
Carter proposed legislation that would impose limits both on
hospital-based capital spending and on hospitals' overall revenue
collection.[12] The plan was defeated by the influential hospital industry, which promised instead to implement a voluntary cost-
containment effort. But the voluntary effort failed, and costs were
soon rising faster than ever.[13]

Congress finally responded in the early 1980s: first by authorizing the states to develop new ways of reducing Medicaid payments
to hospitals, and second, in 1983, by revolutionizing the way hospitals were paid for care rendered to Medicare clients. Under the
new Medicare system, hospital reimbursement is determined, in
large part, by the medical diagnosis of the particular patient. No
longer can hospitals receive whatever they bill. Instead, hospitals
receive a set fee per patient, based on diagnosis, not actual care
rendered, and regardless of the length of time the patient stays in
the hospital.

Why did Congress change course and adopt in 1983 what it had
rejected in 1979? Why did it adopt a regulatory cost-containment
program under an anti-regulation Republican president, Ronald
Reagan, shortly after it rejected an arguably less burdensome regulatory regime proposed by a Democrat, Jimmy Carter? Political
scientist Lawrence D. Brown points to three factors.[14] First, by the
early 1980s, rising hospital costs had shifted (in the eyes of most
health care policymakers) from a problem to a crisis, particularly
given the nation's rising debt. Second, the industry-led voluntary

cost-containment effort had failed (or as Brown puts it, there was an "authoritative discrediting of nonfederal solutions, especially market solutions").[15] Third, there was an emerging consensus on a regulatory approach: hospital rate setting was working well in a number of states and seemed ready for the national stage.

For all of these reasons, the federal government in 1983 dramatically increased its effort to reduce federal health care costs. The effort worked. The rate of growth in Medicare expenditures declined significantly. Between 1973 and 1982, for example, Medicare spending increased on average 19.2 percent annually; between 1983 and 1992, however, the average annual increase fell to 10.2 percent.[16]

With Medicare reimbursement declining, hospitals increased their efforts to shift costs to other payers. Hospitals began to pad bills submitted to private insurance companies to make up for below cost Medicare and Medicaid payments. As a result, private insurers today pay on average 129 percent of the actual costs incurred by their insured clients.[17] Nursing homes, private physicians, and other health care providers did likewise. In turn, private insurance companies both raised premiums (to pay for the increased payouts) and marketed their product more selectively, denying coverage to high-risk individuals (such as persons with preexisting medical conditions or persons employed in high-risk occupations). These insurance practices raised the nation's health care bill and simultaneously increased the number of the uninsured.

Around this same time (the mid-1980s), health care economists were persuading many large employers that they needed not only to stop paying padded medical bills, but to begin cost-containment initiatives of their own. The economists argued that soaring medical costs were due largely to a system in which doctors provide unnecessary services (because they're paid a separate fee for every service they perform) and consumers don't care (because the bill is paid by a third-party insurer). The economists proposed managed care as the solution, noting that such systems generally give a health plan a set fee per client, regardless of the actual cost of the clients care.[18] Much of the private sector was convinced, and the number of Americans in managed care organizations began to rise sharply. In mid-1993, for example, over 24 percent of privately insured Americans below the age of sixty-five were enrolled in HMOs.[19]

To be sure, many of the newer managed care organizations are not particularly good at managing care or at keeping costs down. This is particularly true of the loosely organized networks of providers and insurers that today dominate much of the managed care market. But if the actual cost effectiveness of managed care remains unclear,[20] the popularity of the approach continues to increase.

By the late 1980s, for example, state Medicaid officials across the nation had joined the managed care bandwagon. The popularity of Medicaid managed care was easy to explain. With Medicaid costs increasing nearly 30 percent annually, there was enormous pressure to cut costs, but few options for doing so. States could cut program eligibility, but there was a nationwide recession, and the program covered less than 50 percent of the poor anyway.[21] States could cut benefits, but even "easy" cuts in, for example, podiatry and chiropractic tend to save little yet generate intense political heat. States could cut provider reimbursement, but, not only do hospitals and nursing homes contest in court any proposed cutbacks, payment often is already so low as to jeopardize access for enrollees. The only plausible alternative, according to many state officials, was to promote more cost-effective health care, and the strategy of choice was managed care. As a result, the number of Medicaid clients in managed care grew from 750,000 in 1983 (3 percent of all enrollees) to 7.8 million in 1994 (23 percent of all enrollees).[22]

The movement toward managed care, along with the changed Medicare reimbursement methodology, signaled a significant change in the U.S. health care system. Health care providers were no longer guaranteed full reimbursement for all services rendered.

For the first time, payers of the health care bill were (occasionally) acting as prudent purchasers.

Not surprisingly, the provider industry (other than the newly emerging HMOs) responded with alarm. Doctors complained that HMOs engaged in excessive micromanagement with their demands for prior authorization for many medical services. Hospitals, especially those that served the poor, argued that reduced reimbursement rates were threatening their financial viability. Drug companies suggested that the changed environment threatened their research and development efforts.

Providers were not alone, however, in demanding help. Consumer advocates noted with alarm that the number of uninsured Americans was rising quickly. For the first time, even middle-class workers were now worried about their insurance status: many knew that by changing jobs they too could join the ranks of the uninsured. Consumer advocates also challenged the movement toward managed care, noting that paying a set fee per patient, regardless of actual care rendered, encourages doctors to skimp on care. Small insurance companies feared the movement toward managed care as well. Too small to form their own managed care networks, these insurers worried about losing market share to large insurance companies, which were busy developing such networks. Finally, and perhaps ironically, even payers (both public and private) continued to complain: the new cost-containment efforts weren't sufficiently containing costs.

With key interest groups suddenly clamoring for reform, Harris Wofford, a liberal Democrat from Pennsylvania, demonstrated the emerging power of the health reform message. Wofford and former Attorney General Richard Thornburgh were competing to replace John Heinz, the Pennsylvania senator who had died in an airplane crash. Thornburgh was heavily favored to win, but Wofford campaigned vigorously on the need for comprehensive health reform and rode the issue to a stunning victory. Shortly thereafter, both Republicans and Democrats were proposing health care reform (though there was never consensus on the form reform should take). Bill Clinton also made health reform a key element in his race for the White House. Soon after his victory, Clinton appointed his wife, Hillary, to produce a comprehensive reform package.

The Only Consensus of the 1993 Debate: Delegate Authority to the States

The 1993 debate over health care reform generally assumed that federal reforms would delegate key decision-making authority to the states. Why the assumption? First, states are deeply entrenched in every facet of health care policy and administration, and the federal government is reluctant to absorb all of these functions. In addition to running Medicaid programs, for example, states supervise much of the nation's private health insurance industry,[23] regulate the quality of care delivered by many medical providers,[24] and, together with local governments, pay over 14 percent of the nation's health care bill.[25] Each state also operates its own worker-compensation system, medical malpractice system, medical education system, and with local governments, public health system.

Second, state officials themselves have significant political influence, especially if they have a former governor in the White House, and while they lobby for increased funding to offset the fiscal burden of rising Medicaid costs, they also are anxious to retain their authority to set policy, regulate quality, and administer programs.

Third, the states' significant health policy role is not a historical accident: Americans have long had a cultural aversion to centralized government authority, and the United States Constitution itself reflects a distrust of federal authority. There is, for example, a long-standing American belief that grounding domestic policy-making in state and local governments results in a decision-making process that is more democratic than that which occurs in Washington, D.C. Similarly, the United States is an extraordinarily heterogeneous society, and Americans have long believed that public policy should, wherever possible, reflect disparate local needs and conditions. This perception is particularly strong in the health care context, given the localized nature of the health care system. Boston and Boise do not (and should not) have identical health care delivery systems, and national decisionmakers are (arguably) too removed to develop responsive and responsible programs.

To be sure, the Constitution delegates more authority to the federal government than eighteenth century anti-federalists deemed appropriate. Moreover, since the mid-1930s, and the enactment of the New Deal, the federal agenda has grown increasingly large. Nevertheless, the constitutional systems of separation of powers, checks and balances, and federalism reflect both the framers desire for limited government and the concern that "factions" (or what we today might call interest groups) would unduly influence federal policymakers.

Given the numerous veto points any federal legislation must elude, there has developed a long-standing (if informal) congressional tradition of establishing broad (and occasionally unreachable) goals and delegating to others (whether federal bureaucrats, state officials, or even private contractors) the hard tasks of spelling out details and implementing actual programs. While this tradition (sometimes) makes possible the consensus needed to enact major legislation, it (often) results as well in increased tasks for state and local officials. This is particularly true where, as in health care, there is sharp disagreement about how best to solve the underlying problem.

Finally, there is also a widely held policy assumption that state and local autonomy encourages policy innovation; allows state and local officials to test, evaluate, and implement those ideas that "work"; and enables federal officials to correct (or abandon) policy initiatives before devising national blueprints. In the words of former Supreme Court Justice Louis Brandeis, "It is one of the happy incidents of the federal system that a single courageous state

may, if its citizens choose, serve as a laboratory, and try novel social and economic experiments without risk to the rest of the
country."[26]

To be sure, advocates for health policy reform rarely looked to
the states for leadership or guidance prior to the 1980s. On the
contrary, liberals targeted for reform the state-based nature of the
health care system (and the social welfare system more generally).
The concerns about the "commitment, capacity, and progressivety"
of the states resulted from three historical experiences.[27] First, and
foremost, was the legacy of slavery and the recognition that civil
rights advances and progressive social programs came only over the
vigorous objections of southern politicians. During the 1930s,
influential southern congressmen, fearful that welfare programs
might undermine the southern sharecropper economy, fought
hard — and successfully — for state control over the then emerging
public welfare system.[28] Thirty years later, during the civil rights
movement, southern leaders fought even harder, though with less
success, against desegregation. Given this history, and given too
the inadequate and inequitable health care systems found in many
states, few reformers cared to anchor health policy in the various
state capitols.

Reformers and analysts also believed, not without justification, that many state officials were inept, corrupt, or unprepared
to tackle hard policy issues. Most state legislators, for example,
worked part-time, without adequate staff or support, and were
under obligation to the party bosses that put them in office.

Finally, advocates were concerned because, when state officials
did create an activist economic agenda, as they did during the
Progressive Era between 1900 and 1919, they focused on expanding highway systems and improving education — not on creating
new and innovative public welfare programs.[29] State bias against
redistributive programs is hardly surprising, given that those programs not only benefit the poor, a politically unpopular minority,
they also undermine a state's position in the interstate competition
for business.[30]

By the early 1990s, however, even liberal reformers were touting states as the main source of leadership in health policy reform. What happened?

First, health care costs, particularly the cost of Medicaid, began to overwhelm state budgets. In 1988, states spent an average of 10.8 percent of their expenditures on Medicaid; by 1992 that figure increased to 17.1 percent (and in some states the percentage was significantly higher).[31] As a result, states scrambled to develop innovative ways to control Medicaid costs.

Second, although Congress did, during the 1980s, pass important health care legislation, it aimed primarily to lower federal health care costs by slowing Medicare spending. The main federal health care expansions conferred new Medicaid coverage on indigent pregnant women and children, which increased the fiscal pressure on state officials. States had more to do and fewer resources to do it with.

Third, state officials have become better prepared to meet the difficult policy challenge of health care reform. Continuing a trend that began in the 1980s, most state legislators now are full-time policymakers, most legislatures have professional staffs, and most state agencies have attracted capable and committed bureaucrats. Moreover, organizations such as the National Governors' Association have emerged as effective lobbyists on behalf of state interests and have proven to be valuable sources of substantive policy advice and technical assistance.

Fourth, judicial decisions during the 1960s and 1970s required most state legislatures to provide greater representation for urban and minority communities. The pivotal Supreme Court decision is *Reynolds v. Sims,* which held that state legislatures needed to abide by the one-man one-vote principle. Before the decision, rural communities often had legislative representation well in excess of their population. By the early 1980s, the redistricting requirements had brought into the nation's statehouses a small cadre of legislators anxious to expand social welfare programs.

Finally, the politics of health care reform is different from welfare politics. Health care reform is not a response to the concerns of poor persons, but those of the politically influential, from middle-class workers concerned about declining insurance coverage to major corporations concerned about foreign competition. Pressure from these communities, as well as the enormous fiscal stress imposed by Medicaid, has led at least some state officials to enact and implement various reforms.

In this context, as the health reform debate began in early 1993, there were few voices calling for a nationally financed and administered reform package (such as an expanded Medicare). Instead, the leading proposals each delegated significant authority to the states. Consider, first, President Clinton's proposal, which assumed that national health insurance could be financed by savings generated by (managed) competition between rival managed care plans. Who would "manage" the competition? New institutions, called regional health alliances. State officials, however, would decide how many regional health alliances each state would have, the jurisdictional boundaries of each alliance, and whether the alliances would be state agencies or nonprofit organizations. The boundary issue would be particularly important, since well-to-do communities would seek to avoid being grouped with poorer communities. The political fighting over boundaries would be significant, much like the ongoing state battles over election and school districting.[32]

Clinton's reform proposal also required states to assure that all people, especially poor people, had adequate access to a choice of health plans. States (and regional alliances) were permitted to offer health plans financial incentives to expand into medically underserved communities. States also had to certify that participating health plans met minimum quality-of-care standards, were fiscally stable, and had the capacity to provide the entire benefit package. States had to develop and implement a new home care program for the disabled. States had to develop plans to integrate the so-called special populations, such as the mentally ill and substance abusers, into the alliance system. States even had to continue operating Medicaid programs, even though Medicaid clients would be shifted into the new alliance system. The residual Medicaid program would provide clients with those benefits, including nursing home care and personal care, not contained in the basic medical benefit package.

Similarly, those moderates and conservatives who opposed Clinton's plan and proposed instead a less bureaucratic and more market-oriented initiative envisioned also a large state administrative role. Senator Jim Cooper, for example, a moderate Democrat from Tennessee, proposed a voluntary form of managed competition under which employees in small firms could purchase insurance coverage through state established Health Plan Purchasing Cooperatives (or HPPCs). These new administrative entities would presumably offer small firms lowered insurance rates by pooling them together. Moreover, the conservative Republicans who proposed only incremental reforms also supported strengthening states' ability to regulate the private insurance market.

Even those to the left of Clinton generally accepted a large state role. The "single-payer" proposals, for example, introduced by Jim McDermott in the House and by Paul Wellstone in the Senate required states to be the single payer of all health care bills. These proposals were patterned after the Canadian health care system in which the ten Canadian provinces tailor their health care system to local needs while meeting five national criteria: the programs must provide universal, comprehensive, accessible, portable, and publicly administered coverage.[33]

Perhaps the only legislator who fought hard for a more nationalized approach was Pete Stark, a Democratic congressman from California and the chairman of the Health Subcommittee of the House Ways and Means Committee. Stark's idea was to expand Medicare to cover the uninsured. For most of 1993, however, Stark's proposal was buried in the avalanche of reform proposals, emerging only for a negative commentary in the *New York Times*.[34] Finally, in the waning moments of the debate, in August 1994, Stark persuaded the House Ways and Means Committee, and later House Majority Leader Richard Gephardt, to support the Medicare-expansion approach. By that time, however, hope for a comprehensive reform package had disappeared. Shortly thereafter, the 103rd Congress adjourned without enacting any health reform legislation.

National Health Reform Fails: All Eyes Turn to the States

There are several reasons that the health reform movement, which seemed poised for success in early 1993, ended in failure less than a year later. First, the interest-group opposition to the Clinton reform initiative was overwhelming. The insurance industry, for example, fiercely opposed the plan: small insurers worried about their survival in a world of managed competition, and large insurers opposed the proposed premium caps. The small business community was another powerful opponent, arguing strongly against the proposed requirement that all employers provide their employees with health insurance.[35] Even health care providers generally opposed the plan, worrying about the emphasis on managed care and the prospect of reduced income.

While group opposition to the plan was strong, group support was nearly nonexistent. The aged, for example, were already protected by Medicare, and were generally unimpressed with the few perks offered to gain their support.[36] Similarly, large academic health centers, while generally supportive of the goal of universal coverage, opposed the requirement that 55 percent of all first year hospital residents be generalists by 1998.[37] Many big businesses also opposed the plan, even though the employer contributions required by the plan often were less than current payment levels. There was, quite simply, no constituency strongly in favor of reform, other than perhaps the uninsured themselves, and they clearly lacked the political influence of the groups arrayed on the other side.

A second explanation for the failure of reform is rooted in U.S. political culture. Americans have long had a cultural aversion to big government, beginning of course with the colonial opposition to distant rule by the British. More recently, antigovernment feelings have increased significantly over the last twenty-five years as politicians from Richard Nixon to Newt Gingrich have argued that government collects too much in taxes and spends too much on social programs. As the Republican victory in the 1994 congressional elections illustrates, the public today is suspicious of liberal (or moderate) proposals to restructure large sections of the U.S. economy. The public became particularly worried that President Clinton's health reform proposal would simultaneously raise their health insurance premiums, alter their health insurance coverage, and reorganize what was for them a generally successful health care delivery system.

Given this political environment, health care reformers were unable to traverse the difficult institutional maze required of any federal legislation. The United States Constitution, for example, imposes numerous barriers to the enactment and implementation of federal legislation, most obviously the requirement that legislation be approved by the two branches of Congress, signed by the president, and upheld (if challenged) by the courts. By separating governmental powers among these numerous institutions, the framers established a system of checks and balances, reducing the likelihood that any influential interest group can dominate government, but reducing also the likelihood of major federal legislation.

In recent years, the institutional barriers to major federal action have become even more pronounced. The decline in popularity of U.S. political parties, for example, makes it more difficult for congressional leaders to broker political deals. Congressional leaders have been weakened also by the rise in congressional subcommittees, the escalating cost of political campaigns, and the increasing power of television. Members of Congress today cater more to political action committees, and the evening news, than to committee chairpersons.[38] Finally, President Clinton was elected with only 43 percent of the popular vote,[39] hardly a powerful mandate with which to overcome institutional inertia.

Given these institutional barriers, the interest group opposition, and U.S. antigovernment political culture, comprehensive national reform may well have been doomed from the start. Second guessing the Clinton strategy may therefore be a waste of time. Nevertheless, Clinton's decision to propose a complicated intergovernmental reform initiative, which relied upon numerous new state and federal bureaucracies, and which delegated significant policymaking authority to state officials, was both a programmatic and political mistake. The problems with this approach are illustrated by the history of another complicated intergovernmental health insurance program, Medicaid. I now turn to that history.

3

Explaining Medicaid Variation

Introduction to Medicaid

Medicaid, enacted by Congress in 1965, provides government-funded health insurance to more than thirty-three million low-income Americans. Until recently, Medicaid spending, while hardly low, increased at a slower rate than either Medicare or private health insurance.[1] In recent years, however, Medicaid spending has escalated rapidly, growing at a rate far faster than other major payers, increasing from approximately $47 billion in 1987 to $88 billion in 1991 to $131 billion in 1993.[2] These cost increases pose particular burdens for state and local governments, which paid approximately 48 percent of the 1993 Medicaid bill (around $56 billion).[3] Indeed, Medicaid now represents over 17 percent of all state spending, is the second biggest item in the typical state's budget (behind only education expenses), and consumes nearly 50 percent of all new state revenue.[4] Since many state officials blame the cost increases on various federal mandates enacted throughout the 1980s, the movement today to provide states with additional program flexibility is a high state priority.

The proposed decentralization of Medicaid decision making is especially ironic, however, given the enormous discretion states had in shaping their Medicaid programs and the enormous variation in state programs that resulted. How is it that states have had such discretion and developed such disparate programs, and yet complain together that their options today are so limited and discouraging? Why did Medicaid programs evolve and vary as they have? What impact does such variation have on proposed solutions to the health care crisis?

In this chapter, I begin an inquiry into these questions, first by describing in greater detail the variation in state Medicaid programs, then by summarizing several theories that seek to explain that variation, and finally by describing why a comparative case study of the California and New York programs would add to and inform the debate.

The First Medicaid Era, 1965–1983:
State Discretion and Interstate Variation

Medicaid is not a single national program, but a collection of fifty state-administered programs, each providing health insurance to low-income state residents. There are thus two sets of laws governing each Medicaid program. The federal Medicaid statute sets forth the broad rules state programs must follow and the formula by which federal financial participation is determined.[5] State law then determines who actually receives coverage, what medical services are covered, and how much providers of care are to be paid.

From 1965 until the early 1980s, federal Medicaid law contained few detailed requirements, delegating instead broad decision-making authority to the states.[6] States used this discretion to develop extraordinarily diverse programs. Over the last decade, however, Congress has imposed various Medicaid mandates in an effort to make the state programs more uniform and more generous. Later I describe the mandates and their impact on the states (programs today are far more generous but no less varied). First, however, I describe the discretion states originally had, and the interstate variation that resulted. The discussion is organized around three questions: who receives Medicaid benefits (eligibility policy), which medical services are covered (benefits policy), and how much will Medicaid pay for such services (reimbursement policy).

Eligibility Policy

Before 1972, the federal government and the states jointly funded four cash assistance programs: old-age assistance, aid to the blind, aid to the permanently and totally disabled, and aid to families with dependent children. Federal law in turn required Medicaid programs to cover the populations enrolled in these programs. This requirement was less restrictive than it appeared, however, since it was the states themselves that established eligibility criteria for the four cash assistance programs. By controlling cash assistance eligibility, the states also controlled Medicaid eligibility.

In 1972, however, Congress created the Supplemental Security Income (SSI) program, which combined three of the state-administered cash assistance programs (those for the aged, blind and disabled) into a single federally-administered program. This legislation threatened the indirect control states maintained over their Medicaid rolls, especially since federal SSI eligibility criteria are more generous than those of many of the former state-run programs. Some states threatened to opt out of Medicaid rather than cover all SSI recipients. For this reason, Congress granted states the option of covering all SSI recipients *or* covering only those aged, blind or disabled residents who met the state's 1972 eligibility criteria.[7] With this amendment, Congress preserved Medicaid's early emphasis on states' rights.

There are, more than twenty years later, a dozen states that still cover the aged, blind and disabled under their 1972 eligibility standards.[8] There also is still extraordinary variation in Aid to Families with Dependent Children (AFDC) programs (see table 1).

In California, for example, an otherwise eligible family of three with monthly income below $694 can receive AFDC (and thus Medicaid). That same family, living in Alabama, needs income

Table 1. Aid to Families with Dependent Children, Income Eligibility Levels, by State and Territory, January 1992[a][b]

State	Payment standard	State	Payment standard
Alabama	$149	Nebraska	$364
Alaska	924	Nevada	372
Arizona	334	New Hampshire	516
Arkansas	204	New Jersey	424
California	694	New Mexico	324
Colorado	421	New York (Suffolk Co.)[c]	703
Connecticut	680	New York (New York City)[c]	577
Delaware	338	North Carolina	272
District of Columbia	409	North Dakota	401
Florida	303	Ohio	334
Georgia	424	Oklahoma	341
Hawaii	666	Oregon	460
Idaho	315	Pennsylvania[c]	421
Illinois	367	Rhode Island	554
Indiana	288	South Carolina	440
Iowa	426	South Dakota	404
Kansas	422	Tennessee	426
Kentucky	526	Texas	184
Louisiana[c]	190	Utah	537
Maine	573	Vermont[c]	673
Maryland	377	Virginia[c]	354
Massachusetts	539	Washington	531
Michigan (Wayne Co.)[c]	459	West Virginia	249
Minnesota	532	Wisconsin[c]	517
Mississippi	368	Wyoming	360
Missouri	292	Puerto Rico	180
Montana	390	Virgin Islands	240

[a]These calculations assume no child-care expenses and work expenses of $90 per month.

[b]Income level at which Medicaid eligibility ends. Because of the minimum payment rule, actual AFDC benefits may end at a slightly different income level.

[c]In States with differentials, figure shown is for area with highest benefits.

Source: Congressional Research Service, *Medicaid Source Book: Background Data and Analysis* (Washington, D.C.: U.S. Government Printing Office, 1993), pp. 172–173.

below $149 to qualify. Similarly, a three-person family in Indiana needs income below $288 to qualify, while their neighbors in Iowa can have income up to $426. Even border states have similar variation. As a result, the federal mandate that states provide Medicaid coverage to all AFDC recipients does little to encourage national uniformity.

The Medicaid statute does more, however, than prescribe minimum eligibility criteria: it also permits states to provide coverage to people other than cash assistance recipients and to receive federal matching funds for the cost of their care. States can, for example, provide Medicaid benefits to people who meet the categorical requirements for federal cash assistance but have income above the income eligibility levels.[9] Thirty-seven states (including the District of Columbia) had adopted this so-called medically needy option as of early 1992.[10]

In New York City, for example, three-person families with monthly income below $577 are eligible for AFDC (and thus Medicaid), yet otherwise eligible families with income between $577 and $750 are eligible for Medicaid as well.[11] Moreover, New York families with income above $750 can also receive coverage when their medical expenditures effectively reduce their income below the cap.[12] The New York family that earns income of $850 per month and incurs monthly medical bills of $150 can receive Medicaid coverage for $50 of their bill.

The interstate variation in medically needy programs is nearly as striking as the variation in state-administered AFDC programs. In California, for example, a three-person family with monthly income below $934 qualifies for coverage, while that same family in Texas needs income below $267 to qualify. Similarly, a family in Vermont needs income below $900 to qualify, while their neighbors in Maine can have income of no more than $458. Interstate variation is again a defining characteristic (see table 2 for the income eligibility levels in the thirty-seven states that have medically needy programs).

Finally, the interstate variation in Medicaid eligibility is in-

Table 2. Medically Needy Monthly Protected Income Levels, Family Size of One through Four, January 1992

	Family of one	Family of two	Family of three	Family of four
Alabama	NA	—	—	—
Alaska	NA	—	—	—
Arizona	NA	—	—	—
Arkansas	$108	$217	$275	$333
California	600	750	934	1,100
Colorado	NA	—	—	—
Connecticut	473	629	773	908
Delaware	NA	—	—	—
District of Columbia	407	428	545	665
Florida[a]	180	241	303	364
Georgia	208	317	375	442
Hawaii	396	531	666	802
Idaho	NA	—	—	—
Illinois	283	385	492	558
Indiana	NA	—	—	—
Iowa	483	483	566	666
Kansas	422	466	470	488
Kentucky	217	267	308	383
Louisiana	100	192	258	317
Maine	315	341	458	575
Maryland	359	400	442	484
Massachusetts	522	650	775	891
Michigan	408	541	567	593
Minnesota	467	583	709	828
Mississippi	NA	—	—	—
Missouri	NA	—	—	—
Montana	407	417	443	469
Nebraska	392	392	492	584
Nevada	NA	—	—	—
New Hampshire	436	608	616	623
New Jersey	350	433	566	658
New Mexico	NA	—	—	—
New York	509	742	750	850
North Carolina	242	317	367	400
North Dakota	345	400	435	530
Ohio	NA	—	—	—
Oklahoma	284	359	459	567
Oregon	413	526	613	753

Table 2. *Continued*

	Family of one	Family of two	Family of three	Family of four
Pennsylvania	425	442	467	587
Rhode Island	558	600	741	850
South Carolina	225	225	283	341
South Dakota	NA	—	—	—
Tennessee	175	192	250	308
Texas	100	211	267	301
Utah	350	430	536	626
Vermont	758	758	900	1,008
Virginia	250	308	358	400
Washington	458	575	650	725
West Virginia	200	275	290	312
Wisconsin	510	592	689	823
Wyoming	NA	—	—	—

[a]Medically needy program eliminated April 1992.

Note: NA = not applicable, no medically needy program.

Source: Congressional Research Service, *Medicaid Source Book: Background Data and Analysis* (Washington D.C.: U.S. Government Printing Office 1993), pp. 194–195.

creased further by those states that provide Medicaid coverage to various groups even though the federal government refuses to participate in the cost of their care. New York, for example, provides coverage to persons (typically able-bodied adult males) who receive state-funded cash assistance, even though such persons are ineligible for any federal Medicaid assistance. The cost of caring for these individuals is borne entirely by the state (and its local governments). Minnesota and other states have similar programs.

Benefits Policy

Federal Medicaid law divides health care services into three general categories: those that state programs must cover, those that states can cover with federal matching funds, and those that states can cover only at their own expense. This typology provides states with significant discretion when establishing Medicaid benefit packages. Moreover, states even have flexibility with respect to services required by federal law. For example, states can impose a cap on the number of times a beneficiary receives a particular service. States can decide if a surgical procedure is "medically necessary" (and if not, refuse coverage). States can impose nominal cost-sharing requirements. States can even provide different benefits to different beneficiaries (though this usually requires federal permission). In short, the options for states are plentiful, and the result is that no two states offer an identical benefit package.

Consider the benefit package available to those recipients who receive Medicaid automatically because of federal law (such as AFDC clients). These clients are guaranteed twelve basic services:

1. Inpatient hospital services
2. Outpatient hospital services
3. Rural health clinic services
4. Federally qualified health center services
5. Other laboratory and x-ray services
6. Nursing facilities for individuals 21 or older
7. Early and periodic screening, diagnostic, and treatment services for children
8. Family planning services (but not abortions)
9. Physicians' services
10. Home health services for individuals entitled to nursing facility care
11. Nurse-midwife services
12. Nurse practitioner services[13]

Nearly every state, however, imposes some restrictions on the amount of such services available to clients. As of January 1991, for example, twenty-two states limited the number of days of covered inpatient care. The limitations ranged from fifteen days per calendar year in Louisiana to forty-five days in Florida.[14] Similarly, most states limit the number of covered physician visits. Several states, for example, cover only one office visit per month; other states have more or less restrictive policies.[15] Many states also limit prescription drug coverage.[16]

To be sure, state discretion to limit the amount or duration of a covered service is not unfettered. In *Tripp v. Coler* (640 F. Supp. 848 [N.D. Ill. 1986]), for example, the court struck down an Illinois program that determined via a statistical analysis whether a client was "overusing" the health care system. The court rejected the state's reliance on statistics alone (without any consideration of medical need). It also found unconscionable the state's decision to end coverage for an entire family based on a family member's overuse. Moreover, states cannot deny services "solely because of the diagnosis, type of illness or condition" of particular beneficiaries.[17] States cannot, for example, offer dental services to all beneficiaries except those with AIDs. By and large, however, the courts (and the federal regulators) have upheld amount, scope, and duration requirements so long as they do not deprive recipients of meaningful access to needed medical care.[18]

While clearly not insignificant, the interstate variation in the provisions of these required services pales in contrast to the variation in optional benefits. As of late 1991, for example, federal matching funds were available for thirty-one optional benefits (ranging from dental services to eyeglasses to services provided in a Christian Science sanitarium), and states could provide still other benefits at their own expense. Moreover, while every state covers at least some optional services, no two states offer the same package of services. This diversity is illustrated in table 3.

Reimbursement Policy

Medicaid is criticized regularly for having reimbursement policies that favor institutional providers (mainly hospitals and nursing homes) and disfavor community-based primary care providers. The available data supports the charge. In 1993, for example, Medicaid paid approximately 93 percent of its beneficiaries' hospital costs, compared with 89 percent by Medicare, and 129 percent by private insurers.[19] In contrast, Medicaid nationally pays physi-

Table 3. Optional Medicaid Services and Number of States[a] Offering Each Service as of October 1, 1991

Service	State offering service to categorically needy only	States offering service to both categorically and medically needy	Total
Podiatrists' services	12	33	45
Optometrists' services	14	36	50
Chiropractors' services	8	19	27
Other practitioners' services	13	32	45
Private duty nursing	8	20	28
Clinical services	15	40	55
Dental services	12	36	48
Physical therapy	11	31	42
Occupational therapy	8	26	34
Speech, hearing, and language disorder	11	29	40
Prescribed drugs	16	38	54
Dentures	8	31	39
Prosthetic devices	14	38	52
Eyeglasses	16	33	49
Diagnostic services	5	21	26
Screening services	4	19	23
Preventative services	3	20	23
Rehabilitative services	12	33	45
Services for age 65 or older in mental institution:			
A. Inpatient hospital services	14	26	40
B. NF services	11	22	33
ICF services for mentally retarded	21	28	49
Inpatient psychiatric services for under age 21	10	29	39
Christian Science nurses	1	2	3
Christian Science sanitoria	4	11	15
NF for under age 21	20	30	50
Emergency hospital services	14	28	42
Personal care services	9	19	28
Transportation services	14	37	51
Case management services	10	33	43
Hospice services	9	24	33
Respiratory care services	3	11	14

[a]Includes the territories. Thus, maximum number is 56.

Source: Congressional Research Service, *Medicaid Source Book: Background Data and Analysis* (Washington, D.C.: U.S. Government Printing Office, 1993), p. 256.

cians less than 40 percent of the average rate paid by private insurers for an outpatient office visit. The Medicaid rate is only 64 percent of the Medicare rate.[20] Some Medicaid programs pay much less. New York, for example, pays only 16 percent of the rate paid by private insurers.

Medicaid's institutional bias is rooted in reimbursement policies established by Congress during the program's early days. From 1965 to 1981, for example, federal law required states to reimburse hospitals for their (reasonable) costs, a mandate borrowed explicitly from the Medicare program. This federal rule, adopted in response to pressure exerted by the influential hospital industry, represented an important restriction on state policymaking authority. As a result, Medicaid spending on hospital care increased rapidly. The more the hospital industry spent, the greater its Medicaid reimbursement.

To be sure, several states tried to enact hospital cost-containment programs. Connecticut tried to simply ignore the federal law and impose a fiscal cap on increases in hospital reimbursement. The courts quickly declared the state's action to be illegal.[21] Other states persuaded federal officials and later Congress to establish a waiver program, under which states could establish their own methodology for determining a hospital's reasonable costs (as opposed to following the Medicare methodology).[22] One of the first to try was California, which, like Connecticut, attempted to impose caps on increases in hospital reimbursement. Once again, however the courts rejected this approach, finding that the caps deprived hospitals of reasonable cost increases.[23]

Other states, such as Massachusetts and New York, more successfully adopted innovative cost-containment systems. These states adopted a methodology called "rate setting," under which hospitals receive a daily, per-patient fee, regardless of actual costs. The rate would typically be set by taking the hospital's average per-patient cost from some prior year and adjusting it for inflation. These systems not only saved money (by providing less-than-actual-cost reimbursement), they also withstood judicial scrutiny.[24]

Nevertheless, even with hospital costs rising nationwide, relatively few states adopted the rate-setting option. Instead, most followed the inflationary Medicare model. John Holahan and Joel Cohen suggest several reasons for the lack of interest in rate setting.[25] First, many state officials believed rate setting did not work, that it was simply another form of ineffective regulatory micromanagement. Others believed that the approach would work too well, both jeopardizing the fiscal health of hospitals and discouraging hospitals from accepting Medicaid clients. Still others were discouraged by the administrative burden of implementing a waiver program, the political burden of challenging hospitals, and the legal burden of federal litigation. For all of these reasons, between 1965 and 1980, most state Medicaid programs utilized the same hospital reimbursement formula: pay the bills.

States were much less uniform in their reimbursement policies toward other health care providers. Despite the variation, however, institutional providers of all types generally did far better than outpatient physicians and clinics. The nursing home industry provides a good example. Congress considered and rejected the option of requiring states to reimburse nursing homes, like hospitals, for their actual costs.[26] Nursing homes lacked the political influence to overcome the bias in favor of state discretion. Congress required only that nursing home rates be "reasonable," and "consistent with efficiency, economy and quality of care." States, not surprisingly, developed an array of reimbursement mechanisms. Some states, like New York, developed generous reimbursement mechanisms, under which institutions were generally paid their costs. Other states, like California, paid a flat per-patient rate that was often below actual costs. The variation was extreme. In 1991, for example, the average nursing home in New York received $120 per day per Medicaid client, far more than the $65 average rate in California.[27]

During the early 1970s, nursing homes in the less generous states continued to seek federal relief. One route, rarely successful, was the courts. A federal judge in Georgia, for example, rejected a challenge to payment ceilings, holding that states had "great latitude" in developing nursing home reimbursement policies.[28]

Nursing homes were more successful in Congress, which in 1972 required that, effective July 1, 1976, nursing home rates be "cost related" (though not "cost based").[29] Nobody knew, however, what "cost-related" rates meant, least of all the federal regulators at the Department of Health, Education, and Welfare (HEW) in charge of implementing the standard.[30] As a result, HEW didn't even issue regulations implementing the new law until June 30, 1976, the day before the new system was to go into effect. For that reason, HEW gave states an additional eighteen months, until January 1978, to comply.

Nursing home owners in low-paying states challenged HEW's tardiness in court and even won a moral victory (the courts held that HEW lacked the authority to delay implementation of the law for eighteen months).[31] The practical impact of the legal victory was limited, however, both because the courts also held that nursing homes were not entitled to monetary relief[32] and because Congress itself abandoned the "cost-related" requirement in late 1980.[33]

In the end, Congress, HEW, and the courts did not impose a uniform nursing home reimbursement methodology, at least during the 1960s and 1970s. Instead, states had the discretion to develop their own approach, and states exercised their discretion in different ways, ranging from the generous (like New York) to the miserly (like California). Even the low-paying states, however, paid enough to attract nursing home participation in the program. This wasn't so with many noninstitutional providers, such as primary care physicians who often cited low reimbursement as the reason they refused to accept Medicaid patients. Nor was it so for most community health clinics, which relied heavily on Medicaid dollars, but which justifiably complained about low reimbursement.

Consider the private physician and the Medicaid client. Until the 1980s, federal Medicaid law provided states with nearly unfettered discretion to determine physician reimbursement rates.

Given this freedom, many states adopted fee schedules, pursuant to which particular medical services were reimbursed at a standard flat rate. By and large, however, the rates were so low as to effectively discourage physician participation. This was especially true in several large northeastern states, such as New York and New Jersey. Even today, for example, New York pays only $11 for a new patient office visit, the lowest Medicaid rate in the country, a rate equal to only 21 percent of the Medicare office visit rate.[34] As a result, by the early 1980s, less than 45 percent of the state's doctors participated in Medicaid, and 79 percent of those that did billed Medicaid less than $10,000 per year.[35]

Other states, while not as low paying as New York, also paid physicians well below both Medicare and private insurance rates. This was true regardless of whether the state used a fee schedule, like New York, or followed instead the Medicare formula (paying the "customary, prevailing and reasonable" cost of care). The result was a system characterized both by significant interstate variation and by uniformly low rates. While physician participation rates around the country were generally higher than in New York, participation rates were rarely high enough to provide good access to most Medicaid clients. This led many Medicaid clients to rely on hospital emergency rooms as their primary source of care, thereby exacerbating further Medicaid's institutional bias. It also encouraged a small number of doctors to operate so-called Medicaid mills, or outpatient clinics, in which too many beneficiaries were seen far too quickly, often resulting in poor quality care.

To be sure, Medicaid clients weren't always forced to choose between the emergency room and the Medicaid mill. One alternative in many poor communities was federally funded community health centers, which often provided high-quality primary care to low-income populations. The community health centers, however, had their own set of problems with Medicaid. First, many clinics relied on nonphysician providers (such as physician assistants) who were ineligible to receive Medicaid provider reimbursement. Second, many clinics provided care that skirted the boundaries between medical and social services, care that Medicaid programs often refused to finance. Third, community clinic reimbursement, even when available, was generally inadequate.

The Second Medicaid Era, 1984–1992: Federal Mandates, Rising Costs, and Intergovernmental Disputes

Beginning in the mid-1980s, the federal government significantly increased its control over state Medicaid programs. Congress required states to provide coverage to millions of new enrollees, mainly pregnant women and young children. Congress also required states to provide a more comprehensive benefit package. Congress (and the federal courts) even required states to increase reimbursement payments, both to institutional providers and, for the first time, to primary care providers. These federal mandates, added with the general health inflation sweeping the nation, led to unprecedented increases in Medicaid spending. The mandates led also to increased intergovernmental tension as state officials, who still operated fifty extraordinarily varied programs, complained regularly of federal micromanagement.

States responded to the increased federal activity with some creative maneuvers to shift billions in Medicaid costs back to the federal treasury. States also began campaigning for increased discretion and flexibility, a message that by the mid-1990s became a clarion call. Later, I describe this state activity and the new Medicaid era it helped to produce. First, however, I consider the era of federal domination and its impact on each arena of Medicaid policy.

Eligibility Policy

The Medicaid changes enacted in the mid-1980s represented a major shift in federal health care policy. A short history lesson illustrates the point. The story begins in 1949, when Congress defeated President Harry Truman's proposal for national health insurance. The next year, Congress provided federal funds to states to pay for the medical care of welfare recipients. The new program was popular with conservatives (who believed a medical safety net for the poor would undermine arguments for a more comprehensive national reform program) and liberals (who saw it as an incremental expansion that would help many in need). Since that time, Congress has consistently followed this welfare-medicine approach, providing a medical safety net to the "deserving poor" (through programs like Medicaid) while rejecting all claims for a more comprehensive national health insurance system.

By linking Medicaid coverage to welfare status, however, Congress made Medicaid eligibility subject to the vagaries of welfare politics. The interstate variation in AFDC coverage, for example, means interstate variation as well in Medicaid coverage. This welfare connection became increasingly important in 1981, following the election of President Ronald Reagan, when Congress imposed significant restrictions on AFDC eligibility. As a result, between 1980 and 1992, AFDC eligibility standards fell more than 16 percent.[36] In 1980, for example, a three-person family in California needed income below $805 to qualify for AFDC; by 1992, that same family needed income below $663. Similarly, a three-person family in Alabama needed income less than $201 to qualify in 1980; by 1992, the cap was $149.[37]

The AFDC cutbacks meant that by 1983 less than 40 percent of the nation's poor were on Medicaid, fewer than ever before.[38] The Medicaid cutbacks, along with a decline in the number of privately insured, led to a sharp rise in the number of uninsured. This led to a renewed sense of urgency among liberal reformers. The liberals recognized, however, that Medicaid expansions required conservative support. The conservatives, in turn, were willing to expand the medical safety net for pregnant women and children. One explanation is that many anti-abortion conservatives, such as Congressman Henry Hyde of Illinois, linked support for this population with their pro-life agenda. Second, a growing body of literature suggested that covering pregnant women would actually save public funds. Many poor women, for example, deliver low-birth-weight babies because they go without prenatal care. It is far cheaper to provide prenatal care to one hundred pregnant women than it is to pay the medical bills incurred by a single low-birth-weight baby. Third, pregnant women and children are considered more deserving of government aid than are most other poor people. Fourth, the expansions covered many of the working poor, thereby avoiding the polarized politics of the troubled cash assistance programs.

The eligibility expansions for this population first took the form of expanded state options. In 1986, for example, Congress permitted states to cover pregnant women and children under five who had family income below 100 percent of the federal poverty level. Similarly, in 1987 Congress permitted states to cover pregnant women and infants with family income below 185 percent of poverty. In 1988, however, Congress began converting options into requirements, beginning with a mandate that states cover pregnant women and infants with family income below 100 percent of poverty. During the next year, 1989, Congress required states to cover pregnant women and children under seven with family income below 133 percent of poverty. Then, in 1990, Congress required states to phase in coverage for all children under the age of nineteen with family income below 100 percent of poverty. These requirements had a radical impact. After all, the typical adult applicant (other than a pregnant woman) generally needs income below 50 percent of poverty to qualify.

The states' response to the expansion legislation also went through two stages. Early on most states adopted the expansion options, even the southern states that historically had the nation's least generous programs. State officials, particularly in the south, hoped to reduce high rates of infant mortality and low-birth-weight babies and were now able to use federal Medicaid dollars to address the problem. By the late 1980s, however, as Medicaid costs began to rise, state officials often had second thoughts, especially as the options became mandates. The coalition that supported the expansions began to disintegrate, and after 1990 no new mandates were enacted. Nonetheless, the expansions enacted between 1984 and 1990 today remain in law and help explain why Medicaid enrollment moved from approximately 22.3 million in 1988 to over 33 million in 1993.[39]

Benefit Policy

Federal Medicaid law has always given states significant discretion in developing Medicaid benefit packages. There is the minimum benefit package Congress requires, the thirty-one optional benefits the federal government will help pay for, and the optional benefits provided at 100 percent state expense. With so many options, no two states have ever developed the same benefit package. Over the years, Congress has occasionally added new benefits to the required or optional lists. In 1980, for example, Congress required coverage of nurse-midwife services. A decade later, Congress added nurse practitioner services to the mandatory list. These expansions have been incremental and do not by themselves constitute a major change in direction.

In the late 1980s, however, Congress enacted legislation intended to ensure that required services were being delivered appropriately. Much of the focus was on a child health program called Early and Periodic Screening, Diagnostic, and Treatment services (EPSDT), under which states were required to provide screening and treatment services to Medicaid-eligible youngsters. For years, many states had done a poor job of implementing EPSDT programs, and by 1989 only 39 percent of eligible children were participating.[40] That year, Congress mandated that by 1995 participation levels be increased to 80 percent. Congress also required states to pay for problems detected during the screening even if the services needed were not part of the state's benefit package. For example, if a youngster needed glasses, the state had to provide glasses even if glasses were not part of the state's regular Medicaid benefit package.

Congress also enacted a series of nursing home quality reforms that were to take effect October 1, 1990.[41] The reforms required nursing homes throughout the country to meet minimal standards on several counts, from staff/patient ratios to staff training to patients' rights (nursing homes were required to justify, for example, the use of physical and chemical restraints). The reforms also required states to include the cost of complying with the new standards when developing Medicaid reimbursement rates.[42] The law was enacted in response to growing concern about the quality of care provided in nursing homes to Medicaid beneficiaries. The law reflected Congress's increased willingness to impose new requirements on states and to require states to pay at least part of the increased bill.

Reimbursement Policy

Shortly after becoming president, Ronald Reagan persuaded Congress to provide states with increased flexibility in developing hospital and nursing home reimbursement rates. States responded by enacting a host of new reimbursement methodologies. There was increased Medicaid variation, particularly with respect to hospital reimbursement (most states previously had used the Medicare retrospective reimbursement methodology).

By the end of the decade, however, federal courts regularly were holding that states were underpaying hospitals and nursing homes. There was pressure to raise rates. The pressure increased again when Congress required states to provide additional reimbursement to hospitals that served a disproportionate share of low-income people. Congress also required states to increase the reimbursement received by community health centers and certain primary care providers. Provider reimbursement in all states escalated dramatically. But while states all paid more, the variation both in rate methodologies and in actual rates remained. The reimbursement story of the 1980s was thus increased variation and increased payments.

The story begins in 1980 when Congress abandoned the requirement that nursing home reimbursement be "cost related" and adopted a less restrictive standard, known as the Boren Amendment, requiring that nursing home reimbursement be "reasonable and adequate to meet the costs which must be incurred by efficiently and economically operated facilities."[43] States responded by developing a variety of complicated systems, most of which paid nursing homes a flat rate for each client regardless of actual cost (a so-called prospective reimbursement system), but all of which varied in approach and specifics.[44] Some states developed an individual rate for each home based on the home's prior costs. Others developed a daily rate based on the case mix at the home (the more disabled the patient population, the higher the rate). Still others developed a single rate for a group of homes (dividing homes by size and location). Many combined various elements of each approach.

States differed also in how they reimbursed nursing home services that are provided only occasionally (such as physical therapy and drugs): some included these ancillary services in the basic rate, others paid for them separately. States even differed in how they reimbursed capital costs (such as the costs of construction and renovation).

The hospital reimbursement story is similar. In 1981, Congress decided that the Boren Amendment standard should apply to hospital reimbursement as well.[45] No longer were states required to follow Medicare's practice of reimbursing hospitals for their actual costs. States moved quickly to implement alternate systems. In 1980, forty states followed the Medicare actual cost model;[46] by 1991, the number was four.[47] While the specifics of the new systems varied widely, there were four generic types. First were diagnostic resource group (DRG) systems, adopted by twenty-two states,[48] under which patients are classified by diagnosis and hospitals are reimbursed a set amount for each patient.[49] Also popular was rate setting, adopted by sixteen states, under which Medicaid sets a daily rate for all patients regardless of each patient's diagnosis or the hospital's costs. Under a third approach, used in seven states, Medicaid paid actual costs up to a capped budget. Finally, four states negotiated rates with hospitals. The long-standing uniformity in inpatient reimbursement receded into the past.

During the mid-1980s, the courts generally upheld the new hospital and nursing home reimbursement systems against legal challenge. In *Nebraska Health Care Ass'n v. Dunning* (575 F. Supp. 176 [D. Neb. 1983]), for example, the court held that "Congress intended that states set their own reimbursement rates without stifling and expensive oversight." Similarly, in *Mississippi Hosp. Ass'n v. Heckler* (701 F. 2d 511 [11th Cir. 1983]), the court found that "[a] state of limited resources, in the face of federal cutbacks, has adopted a plan to make the most of its Medicaid funds. The plan complies with flexible federal substantive and procedural requirements and cannot be described as arbitrary or capricious."[50]

During the late 1980s, however, the courts abandoned their deferential approach and struck down several state reimbursement systems. In *Amisub (PSL) v. State of Colorado Dept. of Social Services* (879 F. 2d 789 [10th Cir. 1989]), for example, the court voided Colorado's 46 percent across-the-board cut in hospital payments, holding that "[n]o Colorado hospital, no matter how efficiently and economically operated, would be adequately and reasonably reimbursed for inpatient hospital services." Courts in Washington, New York, and Michigan issued similar decisions.[51] The Supreme Court then put its imprimatur on the Boren Amendment challenges, explicitly rejecting the argument that courts should not decide the reasonableness and adequacy of Medicaid rates.[52] The number of judicial challenges soon multiplied. By 1991, two dozen states were defending Boren Amendment challenges. Medicaid directors sometimes raised rates to settle cases. Other times rates were increased by the courts. States abandoned most efforts to control costs by cutting hospital and nursing home rates.

Rising Medicaid payments were due also to the requirement that states provide additional reimbursement to hospitals that serve a disproportionate number of low-income patients. This provision, enacted in 1981, was ignored for years as states made it exceedingly difficult to qualify as a disproportionate share hospital. In 1987, however, Congress set forth national criteria under which hospitals could qualify for payments. Medicaid disproportionate share payments escalated sharply. In 1990, for example, Medicaid nationally spent $902 million on disproportionate share payments; by 1992 the figure was up to $17.4 billion.[53]

The increased spending on hospitals and nursing homes, while significant, was at least consistent with Medicaid's prior history: the program had always reimbursed institutional providers relatively generously. Beginning in the late 1980s, however, Congress also began mandating that Medicaid programs increase payments to certain primary care providers, such as community health centers, that historically had been grossly underpaid. In 1989, for example, Congress required states to pay 100 percent of the reasonable costs incurred by federally funded community health centers. The new rule provided community health centers with significantly increased revenue.[54] Similarly, the 1989 congressional amendments required states to raise payment rates to obstetricians and pediatricians.

The federal reimbursement mandates, enacted in the late 1980s, contributed to the overall rise in Medicaid spending. The mandates did little, however, to reduce the interstate variation in Medicaid reimbursement rates. States that historically had reimbursed generously, now reimbursed very generously. States that had always paid low rates, now paid slightly higher rates. Every state paid more, but every state still paid differently. This conclusion is illustrated by the following three tables. Table 4 sets forth by state the 1989 per diem rates for skilled nursing facilities. Nursing home payment rates varied from $33.24 in Georgia to $173.51 in the District of Columbia. Table 5 sets forth by state the percentage of a hospital's per-patient cost received from Medicaid in 1993. The percentage ranged from 63 percent in Nevada to 231 percent in New Hampshire. Table 6 sets forth by state the average Medicaid (and Medicare) fee for a physician office visit in 1993. In New

Table 4. Medicaid Per Diem Payment Rates for Nursing Facilities, 1989

	Skilled nursing facility (SNF)	Intermediate care facility (ICF)	Combined SNF/ICF rate
Alabama	$47.22	$35.54	
Alaska			$207.77
Arkansas	35.79	34.99	
California	60.26	44.22	
Colorado			54.30
Connecticut	83.86	64.18	
Delaware			65.21
District of Columbia	173.51	90.07	
Florida			61.14
Georgia	33.24	39.31	
Idaho			52.47
Illinois	49.69	39.73	
Indiana	63.70	51.08	
Iowa	83.55	36.89	
Kentucky	62.32	43.78	
Louisiana	42.62	35.91	
Maine	83.07	58.33	
Massachusetts	90.94	58.76	
Michigan			50.78
Minnesota	68.31	50.90	
Missouri	46.95	44.06	
Montana			50.86
Nebraska	61.91	38.56	
Nevada	68.27	46.29	
New Hampshire	126.20	69.00	
New Jersey	73.70	67.31	
New Mexico	85.65	53.09	
New York	112.93	72.08	
North Carolina	61.40	46.33	
North Dakota	53.62	40.99	
Ohio	59.72	53.36	
Oklahoma	54.00	37.00	
Oregon	83.41	55.71	
Pennsylvania	76.36[a]	65.64[a]	
Rhode Island	75.11	65.00	
South Carolina			46.07[b]

Table 4. *Continued*

	Skilled nursing facility (SNF)	*Intermediate care facility (ICF)*	*Combined SNF/ICF rate*
South Dakota	42.17	33.40	
Tennessee	66.88	38.83	
Texas	49.16[c]	36.36[c]	
Utah	52.60	43.65	
Vermont			59.69
Virginia	70.59	51.78	
Wisconsin	57.27	46.24	
Wyoming			53.74

[a]Ceilings for private facilities in the largest urban areas.

[b]Shifted to separate rates for SNF and ICF in 1988; amount shown is the 1989 average of those rates.

[c]Texas changed to a case mix system in April 1989. Rates shown are those used before that date.

Source: Congressional Research Service, *Medicaid Source Book: Background Data and Analysis* (Washington, D.C.: U.S. Government Printing Office, 1993), pp. 339–340.

York, Medicaid paid $11 for an office visit; in California, in contrast, Medicaid paid $46 for a similar visit.

The Third Medicaid Era, 1992–Present: Returning Power to the States

By the early 1990s, Medicaid costs were rising at unprecedented rates, growing from $54.1 billion in 1988 to $131 billion in 1993. State officials blamed the escalating costs largely on the new federal mandates. This explanation, together with a political environment increasingly hostile to federal micromanagement, brought to a halt the enactment of new Medicaid mandates and even led Congress to consider eliminating federal supervision altogether, instead converting Medicaid into a large block grant.

The story behind the rising Medicaid bill is far more complicated than generally understood, however, and cannot be blamed

Table 5. Medicaid Payments as a Percentage of a Hospital's Per Patient Cost, by State, 1993

State	Medicaid	State	Medicaid
National Average	93%	Colorado	89%
New Hampshire	231	Missouri	89
Tennessee	131	Utah	89
South Carolina	124	Minnesota	88
Texas	117	Arizona	88
Maine	116	Rhode Island	88
New Mexico	116	Washington	88
Mississippi	116	Iowa	88
Maryland	109	Hawaii	87
New Jersey	105	Oregon	86
West Virginia	103	Illinois	85
Virginia	103	Massachusetts	83
South Dakota	103	Florida	83
Ohio	102	Wisconsin	81
New York	101	North Carolina	80
Indiana	97	Pennsylvania	79
North Dakota	97	Nebraska	78
California	96	Delaware	77
Montana	92	Vermont	73
Kentucky	91	Kansas	72
Georgia	91	Connecticut	68
Michigan	91	Nevada	63

Note: Ratios were calculated as the payment received from each payer divided by the cost of treating its patients, including both inpatient and outpatient services. These estimates treat state provider taxes as a general expense, which is consistent with Federal rules that require state taxes to be broad-based. Another approach is to view these taxes as an offset to Medicaid payments because they are used to finance care for the Medicaid population. Under this scenario, Medicaid payment to cost ratios would be: California (88 percent), Georgia (83 percent), Illinois (72 percent), Missouri (79 percent), New Hampshire (169 percent), South Carolina (112 percent), and Tennessee (84 percent). Medicare payment to cost ratios would be slightly higher for these states. Data were not available for about half of all community hospitals in 1993, which may affect the accuracy of the values shown. In addition, the sample size was not sufficient to supply results for Alabama, Alaska, Arkansas, District of Columbia, Idaho, Louisiana, Oklahoma, and Wyoming. The U.S. totals were calculated using reported and imputed data for all hospitals in all 50 states and the District of Columbia.

Source: Prospective Payment Assessment Commission, *Medicare and the American Health Care System* (Washington, D.C.: Prospective Payment Assessment Commission, June 1995), p. 133.

Table 6. Medicaid Fees and Average Medicare Payments for Office Visit, New Patient (Level 3), by State, 1993

State	Medicaid	Medicare	Medicaid as percentage of Medicare
Alabama	$24.75 to 2.18	$45.26	55 to 71
Alaska	90.00 to 135.00	63.68	141 to 211
Arizona	57.42	54.80	105
Arkansas	59.00	48.62	121
California	46.00	59.31	78
Colorado	35.00	47.46	74
Connecticut	26.00 to 45.00	56.06	46 to 80
Delaware	34.00	42.69	80
District of Columbia	30.00	48.38	62
Florida	35.00	52.76	66
Georgia	51.24	47.49	108
Hawaii	60.70	60.18	101
Idaho	44.57	45.07	99
Illinois	25.05 to 29.76	48.76	51 to 61
Indiana	33.21	41.27	80
Iowa	29.23 to 33.47	45.57	64 to 73
Kansas	25.00	43.95	57
Kentucky	39.00	45.36	86
Louisiana	36.00	48.07	75
Maine	24.77	45.78	54
Maryland	37.00	47.25	78
Massachusetts	41.00	49.96	82
Michigan	35.89	47.52	76
Minnesota	35.20 to 51.20	47.27	74 to 108
Mississippi	28.48	36.44	78
Missouri	20.00 to 40.00	45.89	44 to 87
Montana	42.33	48.60	87
Nebraska	39.34	37.21	106
Nevada	47.46	57.77	82
New Hampshire	36.00	45.46	79
New Jersey	17.00 to 22.00	51.34	33 to 43
New Mexico	36.02	48.77	74
New York	11.00	52.29	21
North Carolina	47.01	47.83	98
North Dakota	41.00	45.82	89
Ohio	31.21	46.68	67

Table 6. *Continued*

State	Medicaid	Medicare	Medicaid as percentage of Medicare
Oklahoma	34.97	46.94	74
Oregon	40.93	52.62	78
Pennsylvania	20.00 to 25.00	43.42	46 to 58
Rhode Island	18.00	46.06	39
South Carolina	30.00	41.51	72
South Dakota	44.00	41.94	105
Tennessee	40.00	46.60	86
Texas	47.57	46.41	102
Utah	36.85	43.16	85
Vermont	27.00	48.85	55
Virginia	27.00	39.14	69
Washington	43.13 to 63.14	52.74	82 to 120
West Virginia	36.75	45.94	80
Wisconsin	24.37 to 43.35	44.56	55 to 81
Wyoming	50.98	46.48	110

Source: Physician Payment Review Commission, *Annual Report to Congress* (Washington, D.C.: Physician Payment Review Commission, 1994), p. 356.

solely on the new federal mandates. States themselves developed illusory financing schemes that enabled them to generate billions in additional federal Medicaid dollars without spending any new state money. These initiatives usually worked as follows. Hospitals and nursing homes would meet with state officials and demand a rate increase of $10, say from $100 per day per client to $110 (these numbers are used for simplicity). In a state like New York or California, where the states and the federal government split the Medicaid bill fifty-fifty, such an increase would require both levels of government to now pay $55. The providers and the state would then work out a compromise. The state would raise the Medicaid rate to $110, but the providers either would pay a special state tax of $5 or would simply donate $5 to the state treasury. The providers would end up with a $5 rate increase (the $110 Medicaid payment minus the $5 donation) funded entirely by the federal government.[55]

By 1992, states were using an estimated $7 billion in provider donations or provider taxes to generate almost $11 billion in federal dollars.[56] These initiatives, not surprisingly, generated significant intergovernmental tension as federal officials blamed the states for much of the Medicaid cost increase. Congress even enacted legislation (called the Medicaid Voluntary Contribution and Provider-Specific Tax Amendments of 1991) that prohibited additional donation programs and constrained the tax programs as well. The different levels of government could now each blame the other for the rising Medicaid bill.

It is very difficult to quantify the various causes of the rising Medicaid bill. The best effort so far is a 1993 study conducted jointly by researchers at the Urban Institute and the Kaiser Commission on the Future of Medicaid.[57] This study attributes cost increases from 1988 to 1992 to three general factors: expanded enrollment, general health care inflation (outside the control of Medicaid directors), and Medicaid-only inflation (or increases in Medicaid spending independent of general inflationary pressures). The largest factor, accounting for 36 percent of the growth, was expanded enrollment. Interestingly, however, while half of the new enrollees were due to federal mandates to cover additional pregnant women and children, this population accounted for only 9.3 percent of the total spending growth. Newly eligible aged and disabled persons, in contrast, who comprised only a small percentage of the new enrollees, accounted for nearly 22 percent of the overall spending growth.

The Urban Institute study also found that 26 percent of the growth in Medicaid spending was due to general health inflation and 33 percent was due to Medicaid-only inflation.[58] The Medicaid-only inflation is the product of several factors, including a sicker Medicaid population (many of whom had diseases like AIDs that are costly to treat), more intensive use of certain Medicaid benefits (such as EPSDT services), increased provider payments (due to Boren Amendment litigation), and the donation or tax schemes used by many states to generate additional federal Medicaid dollars.

The Urban Institute study did little, however, to calm the finger pointing over Medicaid cost increases. States demanded (and got) a halt to new federal mandates; Congress demanded (and got) a halt to state provider donation programs. Despite these changes, however, intergovernmental tension remains high. The status quo is particularly difficult for state officials, who must now pay the rising Medicaid bill without shifting much of the cost to Washington. This leaves state officials between a rock and a hard place with significant pressure to cut costs but few options for doing so. The only alternative, according to many, is to emphasize managed care, and nearly every state Medicaid program is now doing so.

By mid-1993 some states were striking a new bargain with federal regulators that allowed states to convert their Medicaid population to managed care and used the (hoped for) savings to finance insurance coverage for the uninsured. Tennessee, for example, is now implementing the TennCare program, under which nearly one million Medicaid clients and 450,000 previously uninsured residents are grouped together in a large managed care pool with the federal government and the states sharing the cost of the bill. This model is now so popular that twenty states have proposed such programs to federal officials, and nearly half have been approved.[59] Moreover, these programs even get waivers from some of the more recent federal mandates, such as the requirement that states pay federally funded community health centers 100 percent of their costs.[60]

This movement toward increased state discretion represents a new stage in Medicaid history. The movement may become so strong that Medicaid eventually will become a federal block grant, under which states will receive a fixed amount of federal Medicaid dollars to spend generally as they see fit. The movement is likely to increase the variation in state Medicaid programs even more. Even without additional state discretion, however, the interstate varia-

Table 7. Medicaid Expenditures by State, Fiscal Year 1993

State	Federal and State Medicaid Spending (thousands)	Medicaid Spending per Beneficiary
Alabama	$1,637,242	$3,139
Alaska	295,384	4,539
Arizona	1,365,046	3,379
Arkansas	1,031,148	3,038
California	13,538,038	2,801
Colorado	1,091,709	3,890
Connecticut	2,274,592	6,817
Delaware	252,993	3,670
District of Columbia	686,719	5,710
Florida	4,948,988	2,836
Georgia	2,798,657	2,930
Hawaii	380,668	3,462
Idaho	293,674	2,951
Illinois	4,981,454	3,569
Indiana	2,815,525	4,984
Iowa	987,200	3,413
Kansas	889,666	3,663
Kentucky	1,863,697	3,017
Louisiana	3,493,823	4,651
Maine	855,860	5,070
Maryland	1,960,419	4,409
Massachusetts	4,131,904	5,402
Michigan	4,362,644	3,724
Minnesota	2,167,025	5,093
Mississippi	1,196,475	2,372
Missouri	2,251,606	3,695
Montana	323,271	3,631
Nebraska	564,169	3,426
Nevada	423,447	4,789
New Hampshire	417,627	5,264
New Jersey	4,706,049	5,930
New Mexico	571,200	2,373
New York	19,980,838	7,286
North Carolina	2,896,330	3,224
North Dakota	269,675	4,343
Ohio	5,179,121	3,474
Oklahoma	1,089,730	2,819

Table 7. *Continued*

State	Federal and State Medicaid Spending (thousands)	Medicaid Spending per Beneficiary
Oregon	955,605	2,938
Pennsylvania	5,612,714	4,589
Rhode Island	829,026	4,337
South Carolina	1,682,379	3,576
South Dakota	266,294	3,826
Tennessee	2,675,390	2,943
Texas	7,118,558	3,084
Utah	477,624	3,224
Vermont	255,476	3,171
Virginia	1,791,773	3,111
Washington	2,316,480	3,657
West Virginia	1,200,412	3,459
Wisconsin	2,114,971	4,489
Wyoming	134,793	2,914
Total	126,405,107	
National Average		3,870

[a]Includes payments made to disproportionate share hospitals (DSH). Excludes federal and state administrative costs.

Source: General Accounting Office, "Medicaid: Spending Pressures Drive States Towards Program Reinvention," *GAO/HEHS-95-122* (April 1995), Table 1.1, pp. 18–19.

tion in Medicaid programs remains extreme. Table 7 illustrates the ongoing variation by setting forth each state's total Medicaid expenditures and their Medicaid spending per beneficiary during fiscal year 1993. New York ranks first, spending $7,286 per beneficiary; California ranks forty-eighth, spending $2,801. Similar states still have dissimilar programs.

Explaining Medicaid Variation: The Social Science Literature

There is a social science literature that tries to explain why state welfare policies vary so dramatically. The first theorist to address the issue was V. O. Key in his 1949 book on southern politics.[61] Key argued that states with two active and effective political parties have more generous welfare programs than do single-party states. Campaigns in one-party states focus on personalities not issues, governments rely on patronage not merit, and the poor lose out. This would explain why the south, dominated for decades by the Democratic party, has such limited welfare programs. The theory wasn't limited, however, to the south. Duane Lockard's book on the New England states also suggests that two-party states (Connecticut, Massachusetts, and Rhode Island) have more generous welfare programs than do their one-party counterparts (Maine, New Hampshire, and Vermont).[62] John Fenton's study of several midwestern states produced similar results.[63]

The political party theory was challenged in the early 1960s by a group of political economists who correlated socioeconomic and political data from all fifty states with state expenditures in five welfare programs and claimed that welfare variation is best explained by variation in socioeconomic conditions. Studies conducted by Richard Dawson and James Robinson,[64] and later Thomas R. Dye,[65] suggest that wealthy, urbanized, and industrialized states have more generous programs; poorer and more rural states have more limited policies.

There was also a third group of researchers who argued that variation in state political culture (not party politics or wealth) best explains variation in state welfare programs. Daniel Elazar, for example, claims that states have one of three political cultures.[66] Mississippi, for example, is dominated by a traditionalistic political culture, which views government primarily as a means of maintaining the status quo, and which encourages regressive welfare programs. Minnesota, in contrast, has a moralistic political culture, which sees government as a means of achieving a better community, and which therefore encourages more generous welfare programs. Then there is Pennsylvania, with its individualistic political culture, which believes government's role is to encourage private sector initiatives, and which has a more middle-of-the-road welfare agenda. Even Elazar admits, however, that classifying states by this typology is a difficult task,[67] though he and others continue to try.[68]

For much of the 1970s, most welfare variation researchers lined up in one of the three camps: interparty competition, socioeconomic demographics, or political culture.[69] The research agenda shifted in the early 1980s, however, primarily because of three factors. First, there was a growing sentiment that the effort to declare a winner in the welfare variation debate was doomed to failure. The three theories each had powerful explanatory value. The goal therefore became to quantify the value of each variable. Second, advances in computer technology enabled researchers to develop sophisticated statistical models that could test the relative importance of numerous variables. Researchers even added several new variables to the equation, such as the impact of economic competition between states.[70] Third, researchers began treating separate welfare programs separately: the explanation for AFDC variation may differ from the explanation for Medicaid variation. There was for the first time research that only examined Medicaid.

The effort to separate the study of welfare variation from that of Medicaid variation was complicated, of course, by the close connection between the two programs: Medicaid eligibility depends largely on welfare eligibility, and variation in welfare policy thus means variation in Medicaid policy. Nonetheless, Medicaid politics differs from welfare politics in at least one important way: there are powerful interest groups (medical providers and the aged) with an interest in increased Medicaid spending; in contrast, the nonelderly on welfare are generally politically powerless. Much of the Medicaid research thus tries to evaluate the extent to which Medicaid variation is due to variation in interest-group politics.

The Medicaid variation literature, while still in its infancy, consists of several interesting and important studies. There is hardly a consensus, however, on the influence of interest-group politics on Medicaid spending. Charles Barrilleaux and Mark Miller, for example, argue that as the size of the local medical community increases, overall Medicaid spending decreases.[71] Saundra Schneider argues the opposite: increases in the supply of doctors increases Medicaid spending.[72] Nor is there consensus on the influence of other variables, such as party politics, state income, or political culture. Schneider downplays the importance of wealth and culture, emphasizing instead party politics and program administration. Barrilleaux and Miller disagree, suggesting that wealth and culture are the key variables. Others weigh in with alternate explanations.[73]

This review of the Medicaid variation literature suggests four observations. First, Medicaid politics is even more complicated than welfare politics. The political environment for Medicaid policymaking is both dense and difficult. Second, the worth of using fifty state surveys to explain Medicaid variation is still unclear. The surveys to date have produced inconsistent results. Third, the surveys so far have not even addressed a key issue: the variation between similarly situated states. New York and Alabama, for example, differ significantly in wealth, party politics, political culture, medical supply, and administrative structure. Every theory so far produced can claim to explain Medicaid variation between these two states. New York and California, however, differ only marginally on each of these variables. Why, then, the variation between them? Fourth, the best way to understand variation between similarly situated states is to conduct a comparative case study. The case study enables the researcher to probe deeply into the history of particular programs, thereby uncovering the explanations behind the statistics.

There are surprisingly few case studies that examine Medicaid variation. Perhaps the best so far was done by Malcolm Goggin in an evaluation of the efforts of five states to implement the EPSDT program.[74] Goggin demonstrates that the variation in state implementation is due primarily to variation in the capabilities and personalities of Medicaid bureaucrats and not to the wealth or political culture of the states.

The dearth of Medicaid studies is matched by the few efforts to examine variation in state health care systems more generally. There is very little known about the black box of state health politics. To help fill this gap, this book provides a comparative case study of the Medicaid programs in California and New York. The case study begins with a description of the two states and an overview of their Medicaid programs. The next four chapters then compare the two programs in four policy arenas: nursing home reimbursement, hospital reimbursement, home care, and managed care.

4

The Medicaid Programs in New York and California

Providing a Policy Context

New York has the nation's most expensive Medicaid program. Total program expenditures in fiscal year 1993 were around $20 billion, or $7,286 per beneficiary.[1] California's Medicaid program is also costly, with 1993 expenditures at around $13.5 billion, but the California program spent an average of only $2,801 on each of its beneficiaries, a per-beneficiary spending that ranks forty-eighth among the fifty states.[2] Put differently, New York's per beneficiary spending is triple that of California.

Why does New York spend so much on so few? Why does California spend so little on so many? These are the policy puzzles posed in this comparative case study.

The best answer is that the variation in Medicaid expenditures reflects variation in the policymaking environment in which Medicaid bureaucrats operate. In California, Medicaid bureaucrats are relatively insulated from interest-group politics and can ensure that costs are kept low. Medicaid bureaucrats in New York, in contrast, are influenced significantly by powerful interest groups (especially institutional medical providers and labor unions), most of whom have an interest in generous spending. To be sure, this is not the only explanation for the variation in expenditures. New York's

Medicaid bureaucrats also are better than their California counterparts at shifting general state expenditures into Medicaid expenditures to maximize federal revenue. But the issue of bureaucratic autonomy is key.

The next four chapters demonstrate the importance of bureaucratic autonomy in four areas of Medicaid policy: nursing home reimbursement, home health care, hospital reimbursement and managed care. To provide some context for that discussion, this chapter offers a brief history of the two states and of the two Medicaid programs they administer. The history is important because states have different bureaucratic styles, patterns that influence the administration of many state programs. In California, for example, the ongoing influence of the Progressive Era (especially the period from 1905 to 1920) has encouraged an independent and influential administrative bureaucracy. In New York, in contrast, interest-group politics is far more prevalent, and social welfare bureaucracies have far less autonomy.

California

The Ongoing Influence of the Progressive Era

For much of the nineteenth century, California was a prize pursued by competing colonial powers. Spanish settlers who had colonized California (and Mexico) three hundred years earlier were challenged by both Mexican revolutionaries and westward-moving Americans. Mexico was the first of the challengers to achieve success. Shortly after obtaining their own independence in 1821, Mexico took over California as well. Two decades later, in 1845, the United States offered to buy California, Texas, and New Mexico for the sum of $40 million each. Mexico rejected the offer and the Mexican War soon followed. After three years of war, the United States emerged victorious, and the three territories became American possessions.

The issue of slavery delayed the effort to grant statehood to the three territories, especially after California in 1849 enacted a state constitution that outlawed the practice. Southern states were concerned that California's admission to the Union would upset the balance of power between free states and slave states. Conversely, several northern states worried that Texas and New Mexico would permit slavery thereby tipping the balance in the other direction. The end result, after much negotiation, was the so-called Compromise of 1850, under which California was admitted to the Union as a free state, while in Texas and New Mexico slavery was permitted.[3]

Even before California became a state, however, its population surged, as fortune-seeking young men were lured by the prospect of finding gold. Indeed, the 1848 California Gold Rush considerably changed the state's demographics as many quiet Hispanic communities were transformed into bustling boom towns. Around the same time, the state's economy also prospered, aided by a diverse and largely undeveloped geography, a steady migration of aggressive and upwardly mobile men,[4] and the construction of a transcontinental railroad line. Nonetheless, as in many economic booms, wealth and power were soon concentrated in the hands of a few: in this boom, the elite that emerged were the railroad magnates. Indeed, according to one historian, "There was hardly an office, from the seats in the United States Senate down through the governorship and the courts to the most inconsiderable town office, in which the right man could not do the railroad a service."[5]

Toward the end of the nineteenth century, however, the railroad magnates became increasingly unpopular. Much of the problem had to do with jobs and race. Rather than hiring American workers, the railroad owners had imported thousands of Chinese to build the railroad lines. The railroads then fired the Chinese workers after the lines were built. The initial decision to hire Chinese workers created racial tension, and the tension increased when the large pool of Chinese workers was laid off and joined the general labor pool. The tension was compounded by the state's economic depression in the 1870s. There was anti-Chinese violence in many California communities. There also was a growing anger at the railroad companies themselves and at the political party (the Republicans) the railroad magnates controlled.

California was not the only state with these sorts of political, economic, and racial tensions. There was in nearly every state a host of problems generated by increased urbanization, industrialization, and immigration. The nation was no longer primarily rural and agrarian. As the number of urban poor increased, so too did the demands on government. There were, for example, new public health perils, ranging from unsanitary sewage systems to deadly epidemics. There were unregulated factories (often called sweatshops) in which immigrants worked long hours for low pay in terrible working conditions. There was a minimal safety net for those who couldn't work, couldn't afford medical care, or couldn't find a place to live.

The demographic changes encouraged many advocates to call for an expanded health and welfare system. Government, however, was ill equipped to respond. The U.S. social welfare policy was shaped by the legacy of the English poor laws: local communities were presumed responsible for insuring the welfare of their residents, and only the so-called deserving poor, or those "legitimately" outside the labor market (due to age or disability) were entitled to local relief.[6] Unemployed nonelderly males didn't qualify. At the same time, most local political systems were becoming increasingly corrupt; they were run by tightly organized political machines that distributed welfare and other benefits only to party stalwarts. Patronage politics, not need, was the criteria for aid.

European countries, then dealing with the same set of issues, responded by increasing the social welfare agenda of their national governments. Germany, for example, enacted national health insurance in 1883 in an effort to placate disgruntled workers. Other countries followed the German lead. American reformers, however, generally known as Progressives, split on the issue of expanded federal authority. Some Progressives, such as Teddy Roosevelt, proposed a "New Nationalism," under which national reform legislation (such as national health insurance) would replace the corrupt and ineffective efforts of local political machines. Most Progressives, however, preferred Woodrow Wilson's policy prescription (known as "New Freedom"), which focused on fixing state and local governments, not displacing them.

The effort to fix state and local governments engaged in by the California legislature was equal to that of any state. The leader of the effort was Hiram Johnson, a former prosecuting attorney who became governor in 1910. The political vision motivating Johnson and California's other Progressive leaders was that reform required that policy and administration be separated. Policy should be made directly by the voters, or by politicians reflecting the wishes of voters. Policy then should be implemented by experts, chosen on merit, who worked for independent administrative agencies. This vision was articulated best by national Progressive theoretician Herbert Croly: "[t]he more clear-sighted progressives almost unanimously believe in a body of expert administrative officials — which shall be placed and continued in office in order to devise means for carrying out the official policy of the state, no matter what that policy may be."[7]

An important element of this agenda was legislation designed to reform the public sector. The requirement of a direct primary, for example, made it more difficult for party leaders simply to appoint political candidates in the stereotypical smoke-filled back room. Voters themselves would have the opportunity to decide on the candidates for public office. At the same time, the state established a civil service system to ensure that government jobs were awarded on merit not patronage. The ability of railroad magnates and machine politicians to reward political activity with public employment was thereby reduced (though not eliminated).

The Progressive agenda also produced various measures designed to place policymaking authority directly in the hands of voters. The referendum and initiative, for example, enabled voters themselves to override the wishes or commands of their elected representatives. The ongoing influence of this approach was illustrated in 1978 when California's voters enacted Proposition 13, which significantly reduced property tax assessments and sharply limited government's ability to subsequently raise such taxes. More recently, California voters in 1994 enacted Proposition 166, which declares that undocumented aliens are ineligible for a range of government health and education programs.[8]

California's Progressives enacted as well various laws designed to regulate the workplace activities of the business community. An important part of this agenda was the effort to encourage a safer workplace, especially for women and children. The legislature enacted a child labor law, for example, that regulated the age of the child workforce, as well as the hours they worked and the wages they received. The state also enacted a worker compensation law, under which employers had to pay for the lost wages and medical bills incurred by workers injured on the job. At the same time, the state created several public commissions and administrative agencies (most notably the State Railroad Commission) both to regulate the state's larger industries and to implement the more general regulatory agenda. For the first time, state regulators were reviewing and restraining the rates charged by railroads.

The regulatory system would only work well, however, if the newly created commissions and administrative agencies had significant bureaucratic autonomy. Without such autonomy, the well-heeled regulated industries might well capture the regulatory process and unduly influence agency outcomes. Here again was the overriding Progressive vision: separate policy from administration and vest administrative authority in scientific experts who would implement policy in an unbiased and apolitical fashion.

By the early 1920s, the Progressive movement had lost much of its national influence. The Progressive party itself lost its popularity and was eventually abandoned. To be sure, some parts of the Progressive legacy survive even today, especially the efforts to encourage a safer workplace and a more qualified public workforce. States still operate worker compensation and civil service systems. But the efforts to fix the state and local political process, and to encourage greater citizen involvement in state and local politics, were generally abandoned. In New York, for example, the direct primary, enacted with great fanfare in 1915, was repealed in the early 1920s. New York's machine-styled political parties withstood the Progressive attack and emerged stronger than ever.

The lesson drawn by many Progressive reformers (including the architects of the New Deal) was that the New Nationalists were right: reform efforts should focus on expanding the federal agenda rather than fixing state and local political systems.

Despite these national trends, however, the Progressive legacy in California remains unusually strong. California's residents (and interest groups) still rely heavily on the initiative (and other tools of "direct democracy"), the state's political parties are relatively weak, and most of the state's administrative agencies have significant bureaucratic autonomy. One reason for the ongoing (and atypical) Progressive legacy was a string of governors who espoused (sometimes indirectly) Progressive ideals. Earl Warren, for example, governor from 1942 to 1952, prided himself (and promoted himself) as a nonpartisan leader in the Progressive tradition. Similarly, Pat Brown, the governor from 1958 to 1966, followed a similar nonpartisan and nonideological style.

Ronald Reagan, of course, hardly fit the Progressive tradition, and when he became governor in 1966, some observers predicted the end of an era. After all, Reagan had promised during the campaign to streamline the state's bureaucracy, reduce government spending, and free small business from unnecessary government regulation. Nonetheless, Reagan soon discovered the advantages that come with a powerful bureaucracy. The best lesson would come from Medi-Cal, California's version of Medicaid, enacted by the state legislature in November 1965.

Medi-Cal Politics: The Reagan Influence

Even before Medi-Cal was enacted, California had an unusually generous health care system for the poor, which included a large county hospital system and one of the nation's most generous indigent health insurance programs. Given this history, many state policymakers, especially the Democrats who dominated the state's legislature, hoped the new initiative would expand and strengthen the state's existing medical safety net. After all, federal dollars would now supplement the state and local dollars already in the system.

Expanding the medical safety net was hardly a high priority for Ronald Reagan, however, who had become governor just months after the program was enacted, well before it provided any benefits to beneficiaries. Reagan was a free-market conservative, and an ideological opponent of most government programs for the poor, including Medi-Cal. His health care agenda was to keep Medi-Cal costs low, limit bureaucratic oversight of medical providers, and encourage competition in the health care industry.

Reagan and the legislature each tried hard to control the implementation of Medi-Cal. The first battle was over which state agency would be designated to administer the newly created program. Reagan's predecessor as governor, Pat Brown, had planned to designate the Department of Social Welfare, the welfare bureaucracy that administered California's earlier indigent health care programs, and many legislative Democrats pressed for that result as well. Reagan opposed the choice, primarily because the agency had a reputation as a liberal social services organization. Reagan wanted to create instead a new health care bureaucracy, separate and distinct from the existing social services community, one that would accept and implement his conservative agenda.

As a newly elected and popular chief executive, Reagan won the battle over program administration. The state created a new health care division within the state's parent health and welfare bureaucracy and assigned to it the task of implementing Medi-Cal. The new division, now called the Department of Health Services, became (and still is) the dominant player in the Medi-Cal policy arena. The leadership of the new division, all Reagan appointees, accepted wholeheartedly his programmatic mission.

While the legislative Democrats lost the battle over program administration, they had enacted into law eligibility and benefit coverage requirements that ensured California would have one of the most expansive and comprehensive programs in the country. Medi-Cal's income eligibility criterion, for example, is higher than that of any other state, providing coverage to otherwise eligible families of three with income below $934 per month.[9] This is consistent with the state's generous welfare eligibility rules more generally: the income criteria for participation in the state's Aid to Families with Dependent Children (AFDC) program is the most generous on the U.S. mainland (ranking only behind Alaska).[10]

The Medi-Cal benefit package also is the most generous in the country, covering thirty optional medical services (only Wisconsin offers as many services).[11] Among the covered medical services are full dental and vision coverage, physical and occupational therapy, respiratory care services, and services provided by Christian Science nurses. Only two other states include Christian Science nurse coverage, and only thirteen others cover respiratory care services.

Medi-Cal's generous eligibility and benefit coverage make the program's relatively low expenditures ($2,801 per beneficiary) even more of a policy puzzle. Alabama, for example, also has low program expenditures ($3,139 per beneficiary), but the low cost there is due largely to restrictive eligibility and benefit coverage policies. More specifically, a three-person family in Alabama needs monthly income below $149 to qualify,[12] and the benefit package there covers only fourteen optional benefits.[13] The story in California is obviously quite different.

The puzzle is explained, in large part, by a tale of bureaucratic mission and success. Medi-Cal managers may have little control over program eligibility, but they have unusually broad discretion in setting provider reimbursement rates, and they've used their discretion to keep reimbursement quite low. Medi-Cal managers are able also to carefully review and control beneficiary utilization of the covered benefit package, and here too they've used their discretion to keep utilization quite low. The result is a Medi-Cal program with high numbers of beneficiaries, each entitled to a comprehensive medical benefit package, but each costing a relatively small amount of money.

New York

Liberal Politics and Decentralized Administration

Medicaid politics in New York, like social welfare politics in the state more generally, is shaped by three political constants. First is a tradition of unusually generous programs and services for the poor and medically underserved. New York City, for example, has the nation's largest and oldest public hospital system. The city also provides an array of services for disabled youngsters, homeless people, and others in need that are unmatched by any other municipality. Similarly, New York was an early innovator in welfare policy, enacting one of the nation's first widows' pensions programs (which became a model for New Deal reformers developing the AFDC program).

Second is a pattern of delegating to the state's fifty-eight local social services districts the tasks of administering and implementing most social welfare programs. This pattern is illustrated clearly by the Medicaid program itself, which delegates to the local social services districts both programmatic and fiscal responsibility. When state policymakers decided to encourage Medicaid clients to enroll in managed care organizations, for example, they assigned to the local districts the task of figuring out how to implement the transition. Similarly, local treasuries must pay more than 20 percent of the typical Medicaid bill. This pattern of delegated authority is not limited, however, to Medicaid. Local districts, especially the district of New York City, have significant discretion in administering and implementing welfare, housing, and mental health policy.

The decentralized and fragmented policy environment contributes to the third constant of New York politics, a history of intergovernmental conflict. This history of conflict dates back to the mid–seventeenth century and the disputes between the British farmers who lived in Long Island and Westchester and the Dutch officials who controlled access to New York City's bustling port.[14] The conflicts then were over money (the high cost of access to the port), nationalism (the British versus the Dutch), and lifestyle (the commercial city folk versus the rural farmers).

The downstate-upstate conflict grew during the debates over the ratification of the United States Constitution. George Clinton, New York's first governor, was an upstate farmer and a leader of the forces that opposed ratification (the anti-federalists). Alexander Hamilton, in turn, was a champion of New York City's commercial interests and a leader of the group that supported ratification (the federalists). The two leaders and the two groups competed fiercely, and the state's decision to ratify the Constitution came only after the document was already in force, having been ratified by a sufficient number of other states to make the New York vote moot.[15]

The intergovernmental conflict repeated itself regularly throughout the nineteenth century: New York City Democrats (including immigrants, the urban poor, and the machine politicians) would battle upstate Republicans (typically farmers and businessmen). The legislative balance of power (which generally resided with the Republicans) was threatened in 1890, when New York City expanded its boundaries, doubling its population. Before losing control of the legislature, however, upstate Republicans organized and orchestrated a power-saving constitutional convention in 1894, during which they secured their vise on the legislature by providing upstate counties with proportionately even greater representation.

It wasn't until the mid-1960s, and the height of the civil rights movement that the courts ordered a legislative reapportionment, which eventually enabled New York City Democrats to gain control of one legislative house, the Assembly. Since that time, the Democrats have maintained control of the Assembly, the Republicans have controlled the state Senate, and legislative politics has remained partisan and divided.

Within the state legislature, two men dominate: the Speaker of the Assembly and the Senate majority leader. These legislative leaders appoint all committee chairmen, control all votes taken on the legislative floor, and must agree on most major legislation. Along with the governor, they form an extraordinarily powerful triumvirate. The 1995 New York state budget illustrates this process at work. Newly elected Republican Governor George Pataki promised to encourage a more public budget-making process, to complete the budget on time (by April 1, 1995), and to produce a budget with less spending, lower taxes, and fewer social service programs. The Speaker of the Assembly, New York City Democrat Sheldon Silver, hoped to restrict tax cuts for the middle class and to protect the state's generous social welfare system. The result was a series of long and secret negotiations between Pataki, Silver, and Senate Majority Leader Joseph Bruno; a budget enacted more than two months late (in early June), and a budget bill that contained some tax cuts (targeted to the middle class); many social service cuts (though less draconian than proposed by Pataki); and significantly reduced state aid for New York City.

As in prior years, however, the task of implementing the legislature's social welfare agenda will be delegated largely to the social services districts. Amendments to the Medicaid program, for example, require local districts to expand their Medicaid managed care initiatives and to increase their efforts to reduce home health care costs. This decentralization of authority makes local politics particularly important in the state's social welfare arena, especially New York City politics. After all, more than 70 percent of the state's Medicaid beneficiaries live in New York City.

The policymaking environment in New York City is, however, hard to characterize and regularly changing. During the 1940s and 1950s, for example, Carmen DeSapio and his political machine dominated city politics. The machine then lost its influence in the early 1960s, leaving city politics far more pluralistic. Social service advocates (including labor leaders, legal services lawyers, consumer advocates, religious leaders, social services agencies, and health care providers) did well in the interest-group bargaining, and the city significantly expanded its social service programs.[16]

New York's interest-group liberalism was severely tested by the fiscal crisis in 1975, during which New York City nearly went bankrupt. The fiscal crisis was caused by a variety of factors, including the recession of the early 1970s, rising welfare costs, rising municipal labor costs, and Wall Street's lack of confidence in the city's budget-making process.[17] While the city survived the fiscal crisis, city politics changed dramatically. In 1992, the city even elected a Republican mayor, Rudolph Giuliani, for the first time in nearly twenty years. Giuliani, like his more recent Democratic predecessors (Ed Koch and David Dinkins) has a pro-business economic development agenda. He also stresses the need to reduce the size of the city's social services infrastructure. Nevertheless, Giuliani's efforts are opposed vigorously by an array of still influential interest groups, and the size and scope of New York City's social services infrastructure remains unusually large.

Medicaid Politics in New York

Like California, New York had a generous health care system for the poor even before Medicaid was enacted. Also like California, the system included a large network of public hospitals, as well as an unusually generous indigent health insurance program. Unlike California, however, in the late 1960s New York had an activist Republican governor, Nelson Rockefeller, who was anxious to work with legislative Democrats in fashioning an expansive Medicaid program.

Rockefeller's motivations were threefold. First, he had presidential ambitions, and he hoped that Medicaid would demonstrate his liberal credentials to moderate Democrats. Second, Medicaid promised to provide federal dollars to supplement (or perhaps even replace) state and local expenditures. Third, Rockefeller had a natural inclination to push for big government projects. He was already committed to a massive expansion of the state's university system, to the construction of the World Trade Center, and to a World's Fair in New York. Medicaid seemed just another worthwhile government project.

There was, to be sure, mild partisan sparring over the terms of the new Medicaid program. Rockefeller, for example, initially proposed that a family of four with annual income below $5,700 be eligible for benefits. The Speaker of the Assembly, Democrat Anthony Travia, proposed instead a $6,700 income ceiling. Either proposal, however, would have produced the nation's most generous eligibility criteria. With the debate so framed, and with both sides anxious for a speedy infusion of federal dollars, there was a quickly negotiated compromise: the annual income level for a family of four was set at $6,000.

Another dispute quickly resolved concerned program administration. Rockefeller proposed that the state's Department of Social Welfare be designated as the state agency in charge of the Medicaid program. Assembly Democrats, who viewed Medicaid as health insurance and not welfare, suggested instead the state's Health Department. Once again, however, the eventual legislation split the difference, designating the welfare agency as the "single state agency" accountable to the federal government, but requiring it to delegate administration of "medical" issues (from regulating quality of care to determining provider reimbursement) to the Health Department.

By April 1966, New York had established its Medicaid program. The authorizing legislation required the immediate implementation of the program, even before the state's plan received federal approval. As later historians pointed out, "It was all surprisingly unquestioned and harmonious."[18]

Within just a few weeks, however, the euphoria (and the apparent political consensus) disappeared. Federal officials were especially concerned by New York's approach. With approximately 45 percent of the state's population potentially eligible for Medicaid coverage (eight million persons), the cost to the federal treasury could be exorbitant. Federal officials had estimated that the Medicaid program nationwide would cost the federal treasury an additional $155 million; New York's program alone, however, was expected to require an additional $217 million in federal funds.[19]

County officials were also concerned about the fiscal burden imposed by Medicaid, since the state had required local districts to pay for 25 percent of the program's cost. While New York City, with its large public hospital system, hoped for a Medicaid windfall (with federal funds replacing city funds), most other counties quickly recognized the large Medicaid payments they would soon be paying. Even New York City officials eventually realized that their hope for a fiscal windfall was unrealistic.

Physicians too made clear their opposition to the new Medicaid program. Many felt sandbagged by a legislative process that moved rapidly and seemed one-sided. Physicians also expressed outrage at the Medicaid fee schedules established for outpatient services. While New York's institutional providers did very well under Medicaid, office-based doctors did miserably. Even today, New York pays the lowest rates in the country for regular physician office visits. The state apparently was willing to accept that few physicians with mainstream practices would also accept Medicaid clients. Not surprisingly, long simmering fears about government regulation and "socialized medicine" reappeared quickly.

In an effort to defuse the conflict, Rockefeller ordered "post-passage" hearings on the merits of the new program. The hearings, held in May 1966, were dominated by program opponents who urged various restrictions and cutbacks.[20] Rockefeller and the legislative Democrats deflected the growing pressure, and the program remained unchanged through the rest of 1966. Moreover, in early 1967, the state even implemented a major effort to enroll more New Yorkers in the program. By late 1967, there were approximately 3.5 million Medicaid beneficiaries statewide.[21]

Federal officials, however, remained anxious to scale back New York's unexpectedly costly program. The result was a 1967 amendment to the Medicaid statute, under which federal Medicaid funds could be spent only on behalf of beneficiaries with income below 133.3 percent of the state's AFDC income eligibility level.[22] Since only New York had Medicaid eligibility levels above the 133.3 percent level, the congressional message to New York policymakers was not hard to decipher.

The threat of reduced federal aid prompted New York policymakers to act. In 1968, the state reduced the annual income eligibility cap for a family of four to $5,300, and in 1969 the cap was reduced again, this time to $5,000. The cutbacks had an immediate and dramatic effect: by late 1969, more than a million New Yorkers were removed from the Medicaid rolls. To be sure, even with the cutbacks, New York's program still contained relatively generous income eligibility criteria. As of 1992, for example, the state's income cap for Medicaid eligibility was the fifth highest in the nation (behind California, Vermont, Massachusetts, and Connecticut).[23] But the possibility that Medicaid in New York would become the public piece in a *de facto* universal insurance program was eliminated.

At the same time, New York's Medicaid benefit package, while comprehensive, was not a national leader. As of 1991, for example, the state provided twenty-six optional medical benefits, which tied it (and six other states) for eighth in the country. Unlike California, New York does not cover chiropractic care, respiratory care, or services provided by Christian Science nurses.

Despite its rather unremarkable eligibility and benefit coverage criteria, New York's program has by far the nation's highest per-beneficiary costs, spending at a level that nearly doubles the national average.[24] As in California, the Medicaid puzzle is best explained by a tale of politics and administration. Unlike California, however, where the story is one of bureaucratic autonomy and low costs, the story in New York is one of an extraordinarily fragmented and decentralized policymaking environment, in which nearly all the key players (including institutional medical providers, labor leaders, and consumer advocates) have an interest in encouraging higher spending and the influence to achieve their goals. This story is illustrated clearly in the four case study chapters that follow.

5

Paying for the Institutionalized Aged: Lessons from Nursing Home Policy

Medicaid and the Nursing Home Industry

Before the New Deal, there were few institutions for the aged. Instead, old people who were unable to live independently typically moved in with their grown children. Since there was, in those years, a relatively small time lag between disability and death,[1] such stays were usually for no more than two to three years. Moreover, with a society far less mobile than today, with few women in the workforce, and with a far younger population,[2] the logistics of such stays were generally manageable.

Inevitably, however, there were many aged persons without a place to stay and without an adequate family support system. The choices for this population were limited. One option, for those who could afford it, was to move into the extra bedroom of a family looking to supplement their income (the so-called mom and pop retirement home). Another option, for a lucky few, was a small number of charitable private homes for the aged, usually operated by immigrant self-help groups.[3] For the majority of the poor, however, the only choice was the local poorhouse, or almshouse. In 1923, for example, 70 percent of the nation's almshouse residents (about 55,000 people) were aged and disabled.[4] These residents endured not only horrific living conditions, but a strong social stigma as well.

The New Deal did little to improve the fortunes of the institutionalized aged. To be sure, the enactment of the Old Age Assistance (OAA) program provided cash benefits to many of the indigent aged, including those few persons who resided in privately run homes for the aged. But Congress also decided that persons residing in the local poorhouses (or in any other "public institution") could not receive federal assistance.[5] After all, these persons were already cared for by a different level of government. Not surprisingly, however, the OAA funding restrictions contributed to the decline of the poorhouse system, thereby reducing even further the options for those without a place to live.

The problem worsened during the 1940s as the demographics of U.S. society began to change. Not only were more and more Americans living longer,[6] society was becoming increasingly urbanized and industrialized as well. In this more mobile and rootless society, families were less able (or willing) to care for and shelter the aged. There was, indeed, a growing crisis: the stock of old age homes was lagging far behind the need. The crisis was particularly severe for the aged who were chronically ill, given the paucity of medically equipped nursing facilities.

For a short time, in response to the crisis, general hospitals were used to house aged persons with chronic illnesses.[7] But with hospitals evolving into specialized medical centers for the acutely ill, this stop-gap measure was short lived. Indeed, by the late 1940s, hospital officials were pressuring patients with chronic illnesses to find alternate living situations.

Eventually, in the 1950s, Congress enacted a series of measures to encourage the growth of medically oriented nursing homes. In 1950, for example, Congress finally permitted residents of public nursing facilities to receive OAA benefits.[8] That same year, Congress established the first system of federal payments to medical vendors (including nursing home operators) who cared for welfare recipients.[9] Several years later, in 1954, Congress amended the Hill-Burton statute to authorize federal funds for the construction of public and nonprofit nursing homes (so long as the home was affiliated with a hospital).[10] And, in 1960, the new Kerr-Mills program authorized federal funding for nursing home care rendered to the elderly poor even if the beneficiaries weren't on public assistance.[11]

Each of these measures encouraged growth in the nursing home industry. Generally speaking, however, the growth was incremental. Then, in 1965, Congress enacted Medicaid. There was, suddenly, a deep-pocket third-party payer for most nursing home care. Medicaid even reimbursed the cost of constructing new nursing homes. As a result, the nation's supply of nursing home beds expanded dramatically, from 300,000 in 1963 to 1.3 million in 1977 to over 1.7 million in 1993.[12]

The nursing home industry remains today extraordinarily dependent on Medicaid reimbursement. There is no other major third-party payer of care. Relatively few Americans have private long-term care insurance, and Medicare's nursing home coverage is minimal.[13] As a result, Medicaid in 1990 funded nearly 45 percent of all nursing home care, individuals themselves paid another 45 percent, and the other payers together paid 10 percent.[14] This purchasing power provides state Medicaid officials (who set reimbursement rates) with enormous leverage, and states exercise their leverage in very different ways. In 1991, for example, a skilled nursing facility in New York received, on average, $120 per day for every Medicaid patient.[15] In California, in contrast, a similarly situated facility received approximately $65 per day.[16] Similarly, a 1990 General Accounting Office report notes that New York spends an average of $11,303 on each aged Medicaid beneficiary; California pays $2,221.[17] In the rest of this chapter, I examine and explain this puzzling outcome.

Policy in New York, 1966–1974:
Pluralism Prompts High Costs

Between 1961 and 1966, nursing homes in New York that accepted welfare clients negotiated reimbursement rates with county social services commissioners.[18] By and large, providers did well in these negotiations, and the typical rate guaranteed reimbursement well above providers' costs.[19] One reason for such successful negotiations was simply supply and demand: with few homes willing (or able) to care for the indigent aged, and with a large number of indigent aged in need of institutionalization, the homes were negotiating from a position of strength.

In 1966, however, with the enactment of Medicaid, the state legislature charged New York's Department of Health with the task of establishing a more uniform reimbursement system. The department decided that Medicaid should pay only for nursing homes' "reasonable costs." Nursing home owners, fearing rate decreases, opposed the new system. Some facilities threatened to stop accepting Medicaid patients. Given the undersupply of nursing home beds, the threat of boycott was taken seriously. State officials, anxious to ensure provider participation in the new Medicaid program, backtracked quickly and allowed nursing homes to receive their cost-plus rates until they could increase their costs to match the rate.[20] The political influence of the industry thus was established early on.

Nursing home owners recognized, of course, the inflationary incentives inherent in a cost-based system: the higher a provider's costs, the higher its reimbursement. For this reason, nursing homes used the interim between the old and the new reimbursement systems to increase their costs significantly. By the time Medicaid officials implemented the new system in 1968, provider costs had surpassed their old negotiated rates. Indeed, Medicaid reimbursement rates were soon escalating dramatically. Between 1967 and 1975, for example, the average Medicaid nursing home rate increased more than 150 percent. By 1974, the average Medicaid rate in a skilled nursing facility was $40.62 per patient per day (and some homes received more than $70 per day). In California, by contrast, the maximum rate then paid to a nursing home was $18.42 per patient per day.[21] But New York was not the only state to adopt a reasonable-cost reimbursement system. Why then was cost inflation in New York so severe? Four factors seem most relevant.

Health Care Unions

Nursing homes in New York pay unusually high wages to their nonprofessional employees.[22] In 1985, for example, a nurse's aide in New York City made on average $8.50 per hour; her counterpart in Los Angeles made $4.48. That same year, a cook in a New York City facility earned on average $10.36 per hour; her counterpart in Los Angeles earned $5.17.[23] These wage differences contribute significantly to the high Medicaid rates in New York. After all, nearly 75 percent of nursing home expenditures are for employee wages.[24] Moreover, the disparity is not accounted for by differences in the local cost of living. The cost of living in Los Angeles is higher. Rather, the best explanation for New York's higher wages is the political influence of its health care unions.

During the 1960s, for example, union officials worked closely with civil rights leaders in an effort to organize New York City's largely minority, nonprofessional, health care workforce.[25] Most of the early organizing efforts were in the city's hospitals, particularly the nonprofit facilities (which did relatively little to hinder union activity). As a result, New York's hospital workers organized sooner and more effectively than did their counterparts around the country.[26] Union officials also began organizing hospital workers and nursing home employees into single bargaining units, enabling nursing home personnel to achieve significant influence and bargaining power.

By the late 1960s, the actual wage negotiations between union leaders and nursing home industry representatives resembled political theater. After all, health care workers' wages are paid, ultimately, by third-party payers, primarily Medicaid. The costs of wage settlements are thus borne largely by the federal government, which was uninvolved in the actual negotiations. At the same time, the parties to the actual negotiations all shared an interest in generous settlements. Industry representatives recognized that wage increases were good business: union leaders were mollified, employees were happy, and industry profit margins were unaffected. New York City's mayor, John Lindsay, who was anxious to improve his shaky relationship with the city's union workforce,[27] was concerned that a union strike could trigger massive race riots.[28] Governor Nelson Rockefeller, then running for president as a moderate Republican, hoped to win votes by providing dramatic wage increases to the union workers (why not, the federal and local governments were picking up 75 percent of the tab).[29] Given this environment, the health care workers were soon receiving generous wage increases: 24 percent in 1966, 25 percent in 1968, and similar increases during the early 1970s.[30] For a workforce long accustomed to sweatshop salaries, the new era offered reason to rejoice.

Interestingly, the large wage increases were inconsistent with the spirit (if not the letter) of New York's Medicaid reimbursement formula. More specifically, state law supposedly limited Medicaid reimbursement of 1968 wages to the 1966 wage amount adjusted for inflation. The negotiated increases clearly exceeded inflation. Nonetheless, Department of Health officials improvised and developed a concept called the "substitute labor price movement" (or "slip-ems") under which negotiated wage increases were substituted for inflation-based increases and were reimbursed in full. Since department officials themselves wrote the reimbursement regulations, they felt entitled to amend them; after all, the increases were purportedly necessary to avoid a political and medical catastrophe (a strike). The real loser was the federal government, which paid half the tab. But federal officials never complained, and wages continued to rise.

Expensive Nonprofit Nursing Homes

Beginning in the late 1960s, New York issued low-interest loans to nonprofit organizations to finance the construction of nearly ninety nursing homes (and over seventeen thousand nursing home beds).[31] The goal was to counteract the business orientation of the rapidly growing nursing home industry. The program was a success: by 1974, 25 percent of the state's eighty-one thousand nursing home beds were owned by nonprofits.[32] (In California, in contrast, for-profit businesses own approximately 90 percent of all nursing home beds, with nearly half of those owned by large nursing home chains.)

New York's newly built nonprofit facilities were elaborate and expensive; construction costs were 50 to 100 percent higher than those incurred by privately built facilities.[33] Moreover, the Medicaid reimbursement rate received by the nonprofits included a generous capital cost component and were thus significantly higher than the rates received by the for-profit facilities. Put simply, the state gave the nonprofits money to build expensive homes and then based Medicaid rates in large part on the high construction costs.

Fraud and Abuse

Significant nursing home fraud and abuse existed in New York in the pre-1975 era. The fraud was attributable, in part, to the cost-based reimbursement system, which encouraged homes to inflate costs so as to inflate reimbursement. Nursing home rates for 1972 and 1973, for example, were calculated by taking costs from 1970 and adjusting them upwards for inflation. This system encouraged facilities to pad their costs in "base years" (like 1970) and minimize their costs (below the inflation trend level) in other years (like 1973). The reimbursement methodology thereby encouraged significant gamesmanship.

There was, in addition, a paucity of Medicaid auditors whose job it was to audit cost reports and report fiscal irregularities. Until the mid-1970s, there were only fourteen auditors for more than eight hundred facilities.[34] Moreover, nursing homes were not penalized if costs were overstated. Instead, facilities that were caught exaggerating costs simply had to pay back the amount above costs. As Bruce Spitz points out, "[t]his effectively allowed the home to take out a 'free loan' from the state by overstating costs and paying back only the principal."[35]

In this environment, nursing home fraud occurred regularly. Indeed, it wasn't until the mid-1970s, when the fraud became front-page news, and the state hired dozens of new auditors, that the extent of the problem became clear. Of course, many owners operated high-quality and extremely reputable facilities. But others engaged in all sorts of financial trickery to inflate their costs (both legally and illegally), particularly their capital costs.

Decentralized Governmental Administration

New York State's Department of Health was not the only governmental bureaucracy involved in the Medicaid reimbursement system. For example, nursing homes were required to submit Medicaid bills to their local social services department. The counties would then pay the bills and submit claims to the state for the state and federal share.[36] But the counties, especially the three counties in New York City, were utterly unprepared to perform this administrative task. There were simply too few people with too few resources to do the job right.[37] City workers generally paid any and all bills, no questions asked, and left efforts to verify and audit to the state. Since, as discussed earlier, the state's Department of Health also had little audit capacity, audits were few.

Because the counties paid the bills, however, they also exercised significant de facto influence over policy. Counties used that authority on occasion in ways helpful to nursing homes, even if it meant stretching and altering legal requirements. For example, nursing homes often complained that Medicaid recipients failed to pay their share of the nursing home bill.[38] In the late 1960s, in an effort to encourage nursing homes to accept Medicaid patients (many of whom were languishing for months in overcrowded public hospitals), New York City officials decided to reimburse homes for the amounts the homes were unable to collect from recipients. This policy, clearly illegal, continued until 1982, when a federal audit uncovered the practice. State officials had long known of the policy but chose not to intervene until ordered to do so by the federal government.

Policy in New York, 1974–1975: Scandals and Budget Crises

In late 1974, the *New York Times* began an extended exposé of New York's nursing home industry.[39] According to the *Times* and the numerous investigators who followed up on the newspaper's allegations,[40] some nursing home owners were stealing millions from the Medicaid program, operating homes that provided scandalously poor care, and using political connections to further their criminal schemes.

Around this same time, both New York City and New York State faced daunting fiscal crises. The city's crisis was particularly acute; in 1975 it nearly went bankrupt.[41] While the state was never in danger of bankruptcy, it too faced a sizable budget deficit, and Governor Hugh Carey decided to slash state spending. Not surprisingly (given the ongoing nursing home scandals), the nursing home portion of the Medicaid budget was an attractive candidate for cutbacks. As a result, state officials enacted a series of nursing home cost-containment measures.

Indeed, for a while it seemed that state officials would actually assume control of the nursing home industry. Every few months there was another dramatic state action, and, rather remarkably, Medicaid payments to nursing homes in 1976 totaled $2 million less than in 1975.[42] First, the Department of Health built up its auditing department, reviewed the books of hundreds of facilities, and uncovered some of the more blatant acts of fraud.[43] Second, it tightened significantly the nursing home reimbursement methodology, so much so that more than 50 percent of all nursing homes saw a rate reduction in 1976. Moreover, the new rates were applied retroactively, thus requiring hundreds of facilities to pay money back to the state.[44] Finally, state officials refused for the first time to sign off on wage increases for health care workers. While the unions called a strike, the effort was short lived and unsuccessful.[45]

Policy in New York, 1977 to the Present: Crises Ease and Pluralism Returns

By mid-1977, the fiscal crises had eased, and the nursing home scandals were no longer front-page news. There was suddenly an opportunity for nursing home owners to revitalize their political fortunes, casting themselves as victims of an overzealous, politically biased, regulatory attack. In pressing these claims, nursing homes were aided by bankers (unhappy about nursing home defaults), union leaders (unhappy with declining wages), and key legislators (unhappy that old friends were in trouble).

The challenge to the cost-containment reforms began slowly, with two issues dominating the agenda. First, nursing home owners argued that the revised capital cost regulations were unfair, particularly since many capital costs approved prior to the 1976 amendments were retroactively declared nonreimbursable. The nursing homes also challenged as imprecise and arbitrary a Department of Health initiative to link Medicaid reimbursement to the quality of care provided in a home.

The state responded to the industry lobbying by convening an executive-legislative task force to revisit the controversial reimbursement amendments. Almost immediately, the task force repealed some of the more draconian reforms, ensuring, for example, that capital costs approved prior to the 1976 amendments were reimbursed.[46] By 1980, the effort to link reimbursement to quality of care was gone as well.[47] Moreover, the state developed an administrative hearing procedure (called a "management assessment") in which nursing homes could argue that their Medicaid rate was insufficient to permit compliance with state rules and regulations. This procedure soon became a vehicle through which nursing homes successfully evaded other provisions of the cost-containment amendments.

Finally, the 1978 labor negotiations confirmed that the cost-containment era was over. Governor Carey, up for reelection in 1979, was anxious to avoid another strike. Union leaders, disappointed by their 1976 defeat, were anxious to produce a generous wage increase. When the negotiations between union officials and industry representatives reached a standstill, Governor Carey stepped in to authorize a 14.5 percent wage increase. The contract was signed, the strike averted, and the Medicaid bill increased.

The declining interest in cost containment did not, however, trigger similar disinterest in quality of care. On the contrary, the scandals encouraged newly formed advocacy groups, such as the Nursing Home Community Coalition of New York, to press hard for strict quality-of-care requirements and for vigorous Department of Health enforcement of those requirements. In 1979, advocates found an ally in David Axelrod, the newly appointed commissioner of the Department of Health. As a result, nursing homes were soon complying with new and rigorous requirements, in areas ranging from worker training to patient assessment to patients' rights. The quality of care in many of New York's nursing homes began to improve. At the same time, however, facility costs were escalating rapidly, and facilities were demanding (and receiving) significant rate increases.

To be sure, both state officials and consumer advocates remained suspicious of excessive industry profits. The first priority, however, was improved quality of care, and lobbyists from the state's two largest nursing home associations argued persuasively that quality improvements were expensive.

There was, however, a growing perception that the system was again veering out of control. Nursing home rates were increasingly established via administrative hearings, and facilities hired consultants, lawyers, and others to show that their true costs were significantly higher than first estimated by the state. This system encouraged inequity, as similarly situated homes fared quite differently in the hearing process. Also, nonprofit nursing homes seemed to do particularly well in the administrative process. Indeed, rates for the nonprofits were, on average, 25 percent higher than for similarly situated for-profit facilities.[48] The nonprofits argued that they earned the higher reimbursement by caring for sicker patients. The proprietaries, however, sharply disputed this claim. At the same time, all nursing homes were increasingly hesitant to admit seriously disabled (and expensive) individuals: the nursing home made far greater profit on the relatively healthy and thus low-cost resident. As a result, seriously disabled persons often languished in general hospital beds. This practice created significant problems.

Not only were such hospital beds needed for other patients, but the cost of hospital care dramatically exceeded that of nursing home care.

By the early 1980s, various political forces were again pressuring the state to reform the nursing home reimbursement system. Consumer advocates, convinced finally that quality of care in most homes had improved, now argued that industry profits were excessive. Lobbyists for the proprietary nursing homes argued that the current system favored the nonprofits (while lobbyists for the nonprofits pointed to the high-cost public facilities as the true bandits). Hospital officials grumbled about chronically disabled individuals spending months (or years) in acute care beds. Proponents of home health care argued that the nursing home reimbursement system encouraged facilities to retain lightly disabled persons who would do better living at home. And state budget bureaucrats complained about rising nursing home costs (the average per diem rate for a skilled nursing facility increased from $49.46 in 1978 to $78.70 in 1983).[49]

In this environment, the state health department developed (with the help of experts at the Rensselaer Polytechnic Institute) a case-mix reimbursement system that would link nursing home payment to the mix of patients within the home (the more disabled the patient population, the higher the reimbursement). Before the new system was implemented, however, it encountered a significant political hurdle. A survey revealed that the prevailing wisdom was wrong — nonprofit nursing homes were not caring for a sicker population than were the proprietaries. Moreover, while the patient population in public nursing homes was unusually sick, public homes' spending was so high that they too would lose under a case-mix system. Lobbyists for the nonprofits, and for the public facilities as well, argued that the new system would jeopardize their financial stability by shifting huge sums of money from them to the proprietaries. New York City officials were especially active in pleading the case for its (high-cost) public facilities.

In response to the political uproar, the Department of Health adopted various policies to ease the transition. High-cost facilities could, for example, receive a reimbursement bonus (or an amount above the figure generated by the case-mix calculation). And the state established a program to transfer millions of dollars from homes that profited under the new system to homes that suffered financial losses.[50] With these additions, the impact of the new system proved to be far less onerous than first feared. To be sure, nursing homes are today admitting a more disabled population, and less sick patients (who presumably should be steered into home health care programs) are now the ones languishing in hospital beds. But Medicaid reimbursement to most nursing homes continues to rise, particularly as homes admit increasing numbers of disabled patients. Moreover, the nursing home industry continues to be quite profitable: a Department of Health survey concluded that the state's 284 for-profit homes generated $163 million in profits in 1992; the 200 nonprofit homes generated a surplus of $37 million; while the 43 public facilities, which showed a net loss of $11 million, generally recouped their losses from their local governments.[51]

The implementation of the case-mix system illustrates nicely the political context of nursing home reimbursement in New York. Nonprofit nursing homes originally supported the new system because they thought it would confirm that they treated the most disabled patients and thus would provide them with even greater reimbursement. When that assumption proved to be inaccurate, they revised their position (and their admission practices) and persuaded state officials to ease the impact of the new system. Advocates too initially supported the new approach, believing it would encourage fairer admission practices and improved quality of care. These advocates now complain that (many) nursing homes are using their increased revenue to increase profit margins rather than patient services.[52] State officials, responsive both to the advocates and to the nursing home industry, continue to push nursing homes to improve quality and pay them well for doing so. The lesson: nursing home reimbursement policy in New York emerges continually from the pulling and tugging of a pluralistic political environment.

Policy in California: Autonomous Officials Keep Costs Low

In 1966, newly elected California Governor Ronald Reagan pressed state officials to develop policies that emphasized Medicaid cost containment. In response, officials implemented a novel but simple approach: decide how much the state would spend on nursing home care and cap spending at that amount, impose minimal regulatory oversight over nursing home behavior, and permit facilities with low costs to make a profit.

To implement this cost-containment policy, however, state officials had to centralize the Medicaid decision-making process. Groups that wield significant political clout in New York (particularly nursing home lobbyists, union officials and client advocates) were generally unable to penetrate the decision-making process in California. Instead, these groups lingered on the periphery, occasionally challenging state actions in court, but more typically adapting and adjusting to state policies.

Consider, first, reimbursement policy in California in the late 1960s and early 1970s. By state law, nursing homes were to be reimbursed for their "reasonable costs." Early on, however, the state's finance department established maximum per diem rates for nursing homes. Facilities received no more than the rate ceiling, regardless of actual costs. Moreover, the finance department, with its emphasis on cost containment, kept the rate ceilings relatively low. In 1971, the maximum rate for a nursing home in California was $14 per day, versus an average of $22.70 in New York.[53]

Unable to influence the administrative bureaucracy informally, California's nursing homes convinced a federal judge to order the state Medicaid agency to hold public hearings on the issue of rate methodology.[54] The agency held the hearings but rejected all requests for a facility-specific reimbursement system, adopting instead an explicitly flat-rate system.[55]

The methodology adopted in 1972, with some minor changes, remains in effect today. The system works as follows. (1) Nursing homes submit cost reports to the Department of Health Services. (2) The department audits the reports and determines the median costs for several classes of facilities (based on size, level of care, and location). (3) The department establishes a reimbursement rate for each class (by taking the median costs for each class from a year earlier and adjusting those figures for inflation). (4) Nursing homes in a particular class receive the same reimbursement rate, regardless of actual costs. If their costs are below the rate, the home keeps the difference as profit. If their costs exceed the rate, the difference represents a loss.[56]

The California system produces relatively low reimbursement rates. In 1980, California ranked thirty-eighth among the states in Medicaid expenditures per nursing home resident.[57] Nearly a decade later, in 1989, California ranked forty-fourth. Also in 1989, California ranked twenty-sixth in rates paid to skilled care facilities, with a rate of $60.26 per day (New York ranked fifth, with a rate of $112.93; the national mean was $70.06).[58] Given this variation, it is hardly surprising that, in 1991, New York's program spent $3.8 billion more on its aged recipients than did California ($5.74 billion to $1.94 billion), even though California had 120,000 more aged beneficiaries.[59]

Not surprisingly, many nursing home owners would prefer a facility-specific system in which homes were reimbursed for their actual costs. Nonetheless, the industry, which is dominated by for-profit facilities, has adjusted by keeping employee wages low and by spending relatively little on efforts to improve patient care.

Consider the wage issue. In California only 15 percent of the nursing home workforce is unionized. Indeed, until the early 1980s, health care unions made only minimal efforts to organize California's nursing home workers. The result is that wages are dramatically lower than in New York, where health care unions represent a potent political force. In 1985, for example, a typical nurse's aide in New York City made $8.50 per hour; in Los Angeles a typical aide earned approximately $4.48 per hour.[60] Nearly a decade later, the entry level salary in California for a nurse's aide was only $4.50 an hour, while the average aide's salary was $6.20. Moreover, the average staff turnover rate in California nursing homes is approximately 90 percent.[61]

Consider also quality of care. For years, patient advocates argued that flat-rate reimbursement systems encourage facilities to spend as little as possible on worker training and patient services, and thereby discourage high-quality care. But state officials (including maverick Governor Jerry Brown) were unwilling to raise reimbursement rates (even if the additional funds were targeted to patient care services). Instead, state regulators and nursing home owners lived by an unwritten agreement: while reimbursement rates were low, regulatory oversight was minimal.

This informal working arrangement was challenged, in 1983, when the Commission on California State Government Organization and Economy (a state oversight agency known generally as the "Little Hoover Commission") issued a highly publicized report detailing both the quality-of-care problems in the state's nursing homes and the state's bureaucratic inattention.[62] California nursing homes were notorious, for example, for being understaffed and for using both physical and chemical restraints to keep patients docile. Moreover, the state's licensing and certification division was itself understaffed, and when state inspectors did find deficiencies and impose penalties, nursing homes were expert at evading and avoiding compliance.

Following the release of the Little Hoover report, the state legislature itself held oversight hearings, and it eventually enacted a new Nursing Home Patient Protection Act. But while the new law imposed minimum quality standards and toughened the penalties for noncompliance, the state Medicaid agency neither increased rates (to enable facilities to meet the new requirements) nor significantly increased its auditing staff (to ensure facility compliance).

Nursing home industry lobbyists, while defending the quality of patient care, now framed their request for a revised reimbursement

system as a patients' rights proposal. Patient advocates, union officials, and liberal legislative staffers allied on this issue with the
industry. Even the state's Auditor General recommended that California adopt a facility-specific cost-based reimbursement system,
arguing that flat-rate systems inevitably encourage poor quality. It
was clear, however, that without the support of the state's Medicaid
bureaucracy and the governor, the coalition's efforts would not
succeed.

In 1987, however, the dynamics of the policy process changed
dramatically for the first time in twenty years. Congress enacted a
series of nursing home quality-of-care reforms that were to take
effect October 1, 1990.[63] The reforms required nursing homes
throughout the country to meet minimal standards on several
counts, from staff/patient ratios to staff training to patients' rights
(nursing homes were required to justify, for example, the use of
physical and chemical restraints). The reforms also required states
to include the cost of complying with the new standards when
developing Medicaid reimbursement rates.[64]

It was soon clear that Congress's actions could undermine California's ability to restrain nursing home costs. Indeed, in January
1990, the California Association of Health Facilities (representing
over eight hundred nursing homes) estimated that California's
nursing homes would spend over $1.3 billion annually to imple-
ment the federal reforms. State officials placed a $400 to $600
million price tag on the implementation process. (Implementing
the reforms in New York, in contrast, was expected to cost less than
$20 million per year because the state already required its nursing
homes to meet tough quality standards.)[65]

California officials, anxious to avoid higher nursing home costs,
developed a daring strategy: they accepted an important revision
in the state's Medicaid reimbursement formula but conditioned it
upon a federal waiver from the new quality-of-care requirements.
Specifically, the state's executive branch supported a legislative
amendment (sponsored by nursing home owners, patient advo-

cates, and union leaders) that would provide nursing homes with an additional $100 million per year to be spent on direct patient care services. However, the legislation also contained "poison pill" language (opposed by the key interest groups): if in 1991 or 1992 the federal government or any court required California to spend money complying with the federal reforms, the new reimbursement scheme would be voided.[66]

State officials then began a vigorous lobbying campaign to persuade the Health Care Financing Administration (HCFA) or Congress to grant the state a waiver from the federal quality-of-care reforms. This effort was particularly intriguing because the primary sponsor of the federal reforms was a Democratic congressman from Los Angeles, Henry Waxman. The goal was to persuade Waxman, and others, that HCFA was interpreting the congressional mandate too expansively. According to this argument, the cost (in time, paperwork, and money) of the new reforms (as interpreted by HCFA) clearly outweighed any benefit in patient outcomes.

Not surprisingly, Waxman was unpersuaded, and legal services lawyers challenged in court the state's failure to implement the reform legislation. A federal judge then issued an injunction ordering state officials to comply with the new law. Despite the judicial decision, state officials were not ready to concede defeat, although they did void the 1990 state legislation that would have provided California's nursing homes with an additional $100 million in reimbursement. At the same time, the state commenced its own lawsuit against HCFA, challenging as unlawful HCFA's interpretation of the reform legislation. HCFA responded by sending 111 (of the 139) federal nursing home inspectors to the state to ensure nursing home compliance with the new law (normally state inspectors are charged with that task). HCFA also withheld $24 million in federal reimbursement to penalize the state for its noncompliance.

While the HCFA officials talked tough, and while the state's lawsuit was pending, newly elected Governor Pete Wilson made a personal appeal to President George Bush,[67] convincing the president to overrule his federal regulators: on March 11, 1991, HCFA suddenly agreed that its "interpretative guidelines" were not mandatory, that it would consider more carefully California's objections to the guidelines themselves, and that California could delay its implementation of the reform legislation pending the "new look."[68]

With this federal concession, the dispute moved back to the courts as legal services advocates challenged the HCFA retreat. Some time later, after much political and judicial maneuvering, the court again ordered the state to comply with the federal law (as interpreted by HCFA), rendering moot HCFA's (half-hearted) argument to the contrary.[69] Following this decision, the state (finally) agreed to begin implementation.

The remaining question, however, was whether the new requirements would lead to dramatic increases in Medicaid expenditures. After all, the industry had estimated the cost of implementation at $1 billion, and the state had estimated half a billion. But with implementation now underway, state officials (not surprisingly) were suddenly downplaying the cost of the new law, and refusing to grant any significant reimbursement increases. The issue again moved to the courts, as the nursing homes alleged that the state was violating federal reimbursement requirements. In July 1993, however, the industry and the state settled: nursing homes would receive $2 per bed per day to comply with the federal quality-of-care reforms. The estimated cost to the state: $49 million in fiscal year 1994.[70]

It may be that the nursing home industry and the state both grossly overestimated the cost of the new federal reforms. Or perhaps state officials are inadequately enforcing the new requirements (as patient advocates today insist). Or maybe the state is simply underpaying the state's nursing home facilities. The truth probably lies somewhere in between. What is quite clear, however, is that California officials are fighting to maintain their firm hold on Medicaid expenditures on nursing homes.

Policy in New York and California: Bureaucratic Variation Produces Program Variation

This chapter began with a question: Why does Medicaid in New York pay nursing homes almost twice as much as Medicaid in California? The subsequent examination of the two states reveals a two-fold answer. First, California's Medicaid bureaucrats have more discretion to implement policy than do their counterparts in New York. Key interest groups (including union officials, nursing home owners, and client advocates) are more influential in New York than in California. Second, California's Medicaid bureaucrats have used their discretion to implement a cost containment regime. The result is the flat rate reimbursement system combined with the historically low flat rates. In New York, by contrast, health care unions have produced relatively high wages for their members, owners of nonprofit nursing homes have used low-interest state loans to build elaborate and expensive facilities, and consumer advocates have persuaded state officials to implement a rigorous set of quality-of-care regulations.

This is not to suggest, of course, that interest groups in California are irrelevant or that state bureaucrats in New York are ineffectual. During the mid-1970s, for example, New York regulators demonstrated their ability to control nursing home costs. The implementation of the case-mix reimbursement system in the 1980s also required significant administrative capacity. At the same time, consumer advocates in California used litigation to require the state to implement federal quality-of-care standards, and the nursing home industry bargained with state officials over a rate increase to pay for the new standards.

On the whole, however, the dominant pattern in New York is one of pluralism and high cost, while the pattern in California tilts toward bureaucratic discretion and low cost. Variation in policy-making environments produces variation in program outcomes.

6

Alternatives to Institutionalization: Lessons from Home Care Policy

Home Care and Public Policy

There is a growing demand for home health care services in the United States. The population of older Americans is expanding, the disabled community increasingly asserts a "right" to home care, hospitals are encouraged by insurers to minimize the length of stay of patients, and nursing home beds are reserved increasingly for the severely and chronically ill. At the same time, however, the network of persons able or willing to informally provide in-home services is declining rapidly: the traditional system of informal care relied upon a society far less mobile than today, with few women in the workforce, and with a generally younger population. There is thus increased pressure on health care payers (both public and private) to cover the cost of the home care professional.

Back in the 1950s, for example, public funding of home care services occurred only when a welfare caseworker authorized a chronically ill client to hire a home attendant (usually a friend) to provide a range of supportive services (such as light housekeeping).[1] Welfare spending on such services was quite low. Similarly, during the 1960s and 1970s, Medicaid and Medicare expenditures on home care services remained low: in 1970 for example, Medicare spent $60 million on home care, while Medicaid spent only

$15 million.[2] Beginning in the early 1980s, however, home care expenditures in both programs began to dramatically rise. Medicaid home care spending went from $1.6 billion in fiscal year 1983 to $3.2 billion in 1989 to $5.7 billion in 1991.[3] And Medicaid spending went from $597 million in 1983 to $2.5 billion in 1989 to $4.1 billion in 1991.[4]

But while Medicare and Medicaid both fund increased amounts of home care services, the actual activities funded remain quite different. Medicare follows a strictly medical model: home care workers must be medically trained (such as nurses), and services must be provided under a physician supervised plan. Medicaid, in contrast, funds three separate home care programs: one resembles the Medicare medical model, a second builds on the traditional welfare "home attendant" model, and a third encourages states to offer innovative and unusual services to persons who would otherwise require nursing home care.

To be sure, federal Medicaid law only requires states to have a medical-model home health program (reimbursing medical providers for in-home care provided to recipients eligible for but not receiving nursing home care). But twenty-eight states have "personal care" programs that fund home attendants (and other non-medical personnel) to provide supportive services to the chronically ill,[5] and nearly every state has a federal waiver permitting it to fund innovative home care programs for those at risk of institutionalization.[6]

Not surprisingly, states have adopted radically different approaches in developing and financing Medicaid home care programs. This variation is particularly apparent when comparing New York and California. New York's Medicaid program in 1993 spent nearly $2.1 billion on home care for the poor, with the lions share, $1.6 billion, spent on personal care services.[7] California's program, in contrast, spent $400 million.[8] Similarly, in 1989 only 0.65 percent of California's Medi-Cal recipients received home care, and the state spent an average of only $608 per year on such clients (which placed the state forty-fifth in home care payments per home care client). That same year in New York, in contrast, 5.75 percent of all recipients received Medicaid funded home care, and the program spent an average of $7,983 on each such client.[9]

One explanation for California's low Medi-Cal spending is its decision not to adopt a personal care program until mid-1993, and to instead provide home-attendant services through a social services program entitled In-Home Supportive Services (IHSS). IHSS benefits are funded by the federal government's social services block grant program,[10] and by general state funds, but not by Medicaid funds.[11] Nonetheless, the IHSS program in 1993 spent only $300 million, so California's total payments on home care for the poor was only $700 million, in contrast to New York's $2.1 billion, even though the two states provide services to roughly the same number of beneficiaries.

The goal of this chapter is to explain why New York's home care program is so much more costly than California's. Is this another story of interest-group politics in New York producing an expensive program and autonomous bureaucrats in California keeping costs low? Or is there some other variable that better explains the variation? To answer these questions, this chapter begins with a history and analysis of New York's program, followed by a similar treatment of home care in California.

Policy in New York, 1966–1972: A Welfare Alternative Keeps Medicaid Costs Low

During the late 1960s, Medicaid funded only a small portion of the home care received by New York's aged and disabled. Most home care was funded instead by the Medicare program, which covered primarily short-term services for those recently discharged from hospitals or nursing homes, and by the public assistance system, which paid for home attendants for welfare recipients. While Medicaid at that time covered certain home health services as required by federal law, it neither covered the optional personal care services, nor encouraged innovative home care approaches.

New York's reluctance to expand Medicaid's home care coverage was driven largely by its desire to maximize federal funding. Indeed, the system then in place was funded almost entirely by the federal government, and any Medicaid expansions would only increase the state and local bill. Why? Because the federal government paid 100 percent of the Medicare bill, 75 percent of the public assistance social services bill, but only 50 percent of the Medicaid bill.

There were institutional barriers to an expanded Medicaid home care program as well. For example, the state Department of Health administered Medicaid's small home health care program in a relatively centralized and cost-conscious fashion. Home health care workers were licensed by the Department of Health, supervised by a state-certified home care agency, and paid according to wage schedules established by the state. In contrast, the state Department of Social Services administered the public-assistance home attendant program in an extraordinarily decentralized and fragmented fashion. County welfare officials, welfare caseworkers, and even welfare recipients all had significant influence over the program's implementation and all had an interest in maintaining the status quo.

County welfare officials, for example, determined the wages received by most home attendants. They also established, within broad parameters set by the Department of Social Services, the rules and regulations governing the program. With such authority, local officials could (and did) shape the direction and cost of the program. Not surprisingly, these officials were anxious to retain their authority. But if Medicaid adopted a personal care home attendant program and delegated to the Department of Health the task of administration, local officials would lose most of their control.

Similarly, the system then in place delegated to welfare caseworkers the task of deciding which welfare recipients could receive home attendant services. These workers too were anxious to retain their decision-making authority. Under a Medicaid-funded personal care system, the decision to authorize services would be transferred to a doctor, and the services themselves would be supervised by a registered nurse.

The public-assistance home attendant program also provided welfare recipients with welcome (and uncommon) autonomy. Eligible beneficiaries could hire their own attendants. Oftentimes, they hired friends or neighbors, increasing the likelihood that care was provided with warmth and love. And if it wasn't, the client had the option of firing her attendant and hiring another. To be sure, many recipients were too aged or too disabled to exercise effectively their hiring power, and there were surely abuses of the system as well. Nonetheless, most clients appreciated the unusual opportunity to act as an employer and preferred the informal nature of the system.

Finally, the system offered jobs as home attendants to untrained and unskilled community residents. While the work was hard and poorly paid, it was a job and often a step forward. Many such workers, and advocates on their behalf, would support a Medicaid-funded personal care program only if current workers received the training and the opportunity to keep their jobs. But since nobody could offer such guarantees, the status quo remained the preferred option.

State Department of Social Services officials were aware of the problems created by a decentralized system. They were particularly concerned by the workers' lack of training. But they remained committed to the fragmented and informal program structure,[12] and they were particularly opposed to the adoption of a Medicaid personal care option, fearing it would convert the home attendant program from a welfare program to a health care program, with administration transferred from social workers in the Social Services Department to medical experts in the Health Department. And even those cost-conscious state officials who were troubled by what they saw in the welfare-based home attendant program were reluctant to press too hard for a Medicaid-funded alternative: after all, the federal share of public assistance payments was far higher than its share of the Medicaid bill.

In 1972, however, as part of his "revenue-sharing" proposals, President Richard Nixon persuaded Congress to impose a fiscal cap on the federal program that funded social services (such as home attendants) for welfare clients.[13] The cap threatened to undermine the social services system then in place in New York: the federal contribution would be cut from the original amount of approximately $600 million to around $230 million. The cutbacks prompted state officials to conduct an all-out search for alternate funding streams. One solution, quickly identified, was to convert the public-assistance home attendant program into a Medicaid-funded personal care program. In mid-1973, the New York state legislature enacted this proposal into law.[14]

Medicaid-Funded Home Care Expands, and the System Fragments Further

The legislative decision to adopt a Medicaid-funded personal care program meant that New York now had two very different types of home care programs: a home health program that provided primarily short-term follow-up care to persons discharged from acute care institutions, and a home attendant program that emphasized long-term supportive care to the chronically ill. But there was clear overlap as well, particularly since the decision to shift to Medicaid funding meant that home care services now needed to be medically necessary, prescribed by a physician, and supervised by a nurse. Over time, the functional difference between a personal care home attendant and a home health aide grew blurry. Home attendants, for example, could not only bathe, dress, and feed beneficiaries, they could, if trained, measure and monitor the recipients' physical conditions, assist in exercise programs, and help with prescribed medical equipment.[15]

The two programs might have looked even more alike had the Department of Health received permission to administer the personal care initiative. But the state Department of Social Services, and the other players in the welfare-based home attendant system, were determined to maintain a decentralized, informal, and service-oriented program. These groups pressed for and obtained from the legislature three significant concessions: first, the state Department of Social Services (and not the Department of Health) would administer the new program. Second, local welfare officials would oversee day-to-day program operations. And third, eligible clients would continue to hire their own attendants.

The state's home care environment grew even more fragmented in 1977 when the state legislature required the Department of Health and the Department of Social Services to administer jointly a new home care initiative, called by its sponsors the "nursing home without walls" program. The new program was part of the state's response to the nursing home scandals of the mid-1970s. In addition to imposing (short-term) fiscal controls on nursing home costs and limiting the growth of the nursing home industry (by more rigorously enforcing certificate-of-need regulations), state policymakers were anxious to encourage alternatives to institutionalization, such as home care. The policy assumption was that home care services were more humane and less costly than institutionalization. The nursing home without walls program, for example, permits Medicaid clients at risk of institutionalization to receive in their homes various services not available to other Medicaid clients (so long as the total cost of care is less than 75 percent of the Medicaid nursing home rate).

With this new program, there were now three Medicaid-funded home care programs, each with a different set of rules, regulations, and priorities. Of the three programs, the personal care program generated by far the most controversy, due largely to the extraordinary rate of growth in program expenditures. In 1978, for example, Medicaid expenditures on personal care totaled $140 million; five years later expenditures were up to $457 million. Over that same time period, however, Medicaid expenditures on home health services only went from $30 million to $35 million.[16]

The most persistent and influential critic of New York's personal care program was the federal government. Federal officials were particularly upset by the informal and quasi-medical nature of the program, which in their view was responsible for the rising costs. These officials argued that many personal care services (such as housekeeping and cooking) were insufficiently "medical" to be permissible Medicaid benefits. Federal officials complained also that most home attendants were inadequately trained and supervised.

State Department of Social Services officials who administered the personal care program acknowledged the problem with training and supervision, but correcting the problem was difficult, particularly given the local authority over day-to-day operations. State officials rejected outright, however, all federal efforts to eliminate the nonmedical home attendant benefits. After all, these services represented for many the very heart of the personal care program.

The coverage dispute intensified in early 1979 when federal auditors issued a report declaring many of the nonmedical services ineligible for federal Medicaid reimbursement. State officials challenged that finding before an administrative law judge, insisting that the federal regulations governing the program permitted the coverage. Perhaps surprisingly, the federal judge agreed, and the program survived intact.

Federal officials were not alone, however, in criticizing the personal care program. New York City Council President Paul O'Dwyer, for example, alleged that the personal care industry, much like the nursing home industry, was rife with fraud, abuse, and incompetence.[17] On the one hand, Medicaid payments to home attendants were often extremely late, which created much hardship for a workforce of mostly women who were themselves quite poor. At the same time, however, several housekeeper agencies (which dispatched workers to beneficiaries unable to find their own) were themselves engaging in inappropriate if not illegal activities. The United Neighborhood Services agency in Brooklyn, for example, allegedly used Medicaid funds to establish a summer camp for the children of its workers.[18] While such practices hardly compared to the profit-making schemes of the nursing home barons, their existence illustrated the program's lack of accountability and oversight.

These miniscandals, particularly the administrative delays in processing payments to home attendants, prompted a closer look at the entire industry. Consumer advocates noted that the sixteen thousand home attendants in New York City, who were paid the minimum wage (then $2.90 per hour) plus fifteen cents per hour for meals and transportation, were considered "independent contractors" and were thus ineligible for any government pension, health insurance coverage, or other job benefit.[19] Advocates noted also that as the program grew, fewer and fewer clients hired friends and neighbors, and the bond between client and attendant grew increasingly fragile. As one commentator put it,

> [home attendants] work in thousands of private households isolated from co-workers and supervisory support. Since many clients are poor, workers often have to enter crime-ridden neighborhoods and work in deteriorating tenement housing. They care for people with difficult illnesses . . . and attend to terminally ill and dying clients.[20]

Given these working conditions, and given the publicity generated by the scandals, union leaders began a drive to organize and unionize New York City home attendants. Union leaders demanded not only higher wages, but also a recognition that home attendants were city employees entitled to fringe benefits equivalent to similarly situated public workers. City officials, anxious to avoid the dramatic cost escalation that would accompany such a determination, rejected the argument that home attendants were city workers. But the union activity added additional pressure on a program that now seemed under siege.

Sensing the need to do something dramatic, city officials decided in 1980 to hire nonprofit agencies to administer and supervise the personal care program. No longer would home attendants be classified as "independent contractors." Such workers would now be hired, paid, and trained by private social services agencies, and would receive from them health insurance and other fringe benefits.

The new system benefited most of the key players. Home attendants received better pay, more training, and closer supervision. Clients (presumably) received better care (and if they didn't, there was an organization that would respond to their complaints). Federal auditors were happy that training and supervision was more available. State and local officials were relieved that home attendants were not classified as city employees (thereby entitled to the public sector's even-more-generous benefit package). And all the key players were pleased that the service delivery system remained decentralized.

Perhaps the only group unhappy with the new arrangement was the non-aged, physically disabled community, which generally preferred acting as the de facto employer of their attendant. Many in this community feared a loss of discretion and control as attendants became less accountable to them and more accountable to a social services agency, especially if the agency had little experience in dealing with young disabled persons. In response to these concerns, the disabled community and city officials together established a new nonprofit agency, called Concepts for Independence, which provides attendants to much of the disabled community, thereby increasing the likelihood that disabled clients receive suitable help.

Explaining the High Cost of Medicaid-Funded Home Care

New York's Medicaid program spends far more money on home care than does any other state. The disparity is dramatic. In 1993, for example, New York's program spent nearly $2.1 billion on home care ($1.6 billion of which was on personal care services);[21] nationwide Medicaid expenditures on home care that year were just over $4 billion.[22]

The explanation for New York's high-cost program is understood best as a consequence of a pluralistic policymaking environment in which nearly all of the key players have an interest in program expansion. State policymakers pursue home care as an alternative to institutionalization. Nonprofit home care agencies emphasize service not cost. Union leaders aggressively seek increased compensation for home attendants. Client advocates assert an unbridled "right" to individualized home care services. And a fragmented government bureaucracy acts typically without coordination or consistency, thereby increasing even further overall program costs.

The Open-Ended Entitlement

State officials have long believed that in-home services are cheaper and more humane than institutional care. This policy assumption has led the state to impose strict limits on the construction of new nursing home beds, to develop a nursing home reimbursement methodology that steers the lightly disabled out of institutions and into home care programs, and to develop a hospital reimbursement methodology that encourages hospitals to discharge patients as quickly as possible.

Given this strong state commitment, and given also the strong home care advocacy community, the state never enacted a rigid cap on the number of hours of care a beneficiary can receive per day. The open-ended entitlement created a system in which New York home care clients receive far more hours of care than do their counterparts elsewhere. In 1985, for example, the average home attendant recipient in New York City received over fifty hours of care per week.[23] Moreover, 17 percent of the city's home attendant clients received care twenty-four hours per day, seven days a week,[24] at an average cost of over $90,000 per year per client.[25] This sort of open-ended coverage is not allowed in other states. Texas, for example, which operates the nation's second largest personal care program, limits clients to thirty hours of coverage per week.[26]

The state's Division of the Budget has, for years, proposed legislation to cap the number of hours of permissible home attendant care. By and large, however, such efforts failed miserably. In 1983, for example, in the midst of an economic recession, the Division of the Budget lobbied hard for a ban on twenty-four-hour coverage and a cap on the total number of home care hours each local district could authorize. The bill was fiercely opposed by consumer advocates, social services agencies, local welfare officials, and even many state bureaucrats. These opponents, while unable to block the legislation in its entirety, obtained two key concessions: only twenty-four-hour coverage was barred (so twenty-three hours was permissible), and even twenty-four-hour coverage was allowable for the physically disabled.

Even in its weakened form, however, the bill generated significant controversy. Federal officials were concerned that the distinction drawn between the physically disabled and other home care clients was arbitrary and perhaps illegal. The task of implementing the cap on the number of personal care hours a local district could authorize was extremely difficult. Governor Mario Cuomo, who signed the bill in his first year in office, was having second thoughts. And even the Division of the Budget was hard pressed to support enthusiastically the watered-down legislation that was enacted into law. As a result, in 1984 the personal care cost-containment bill was repealed (only one year after its enactment).

The effort to impose a more rigorous monitoring of home attendant services was revived in 1991 during New York's next budget crisis. The politics during this era were somewhat different given the extraordinary rise in home care costs during the 1980s and given the small number of clients that accounted for a disproportionate share of such expenditures. There were, for example, over 2,400 clients who received annually over $45,000 worth of Medicaid-funded home care services, including 150 or so who received over $100,000 per year.[27] This data made clear that home care was not always cheaper than institutional care. As a result, state officials argued that many of these clients didn't need twenty-four-hour coverage and that others belonged in institutions or group homes.

Given the pressure to pass a home care cost-containment bill, some members of the state's advocacy community, most notably the State Communities Aid Association, agreed to a bill that requires state officials to review closely those Medicaid clients who receive home care services for more than sixty days, and whose home care costs are more than 90 percent of the average cost of a local nursing home.[28] During this review, the burden is on the client to demonstrate either that the high cost is justified or that there is no appropriate alternate level of care available. If the client fails both tests, she or he must either move into the institutional alternative or lose Medicaid coverage.

Not surprisingly, other advocates opposed the 1991 legislation and challenged its legality in court, claiming that its implementation would irreparably harm numerous needy clients. Three years later, in late 1994, the litigation remains unresolved, and the fiscal assessment system has yet to be implemented for most home care clients.[29]

The legislative maneuvering over home care hours resumed again in the 1992 legislative session when Governor Cuomo proposed a cap of 156 hours per month per client. The Republican-dominated state senate proposed an even more restrictive 120-hour cap. But the state assembly, dominated by liberal democrats, never considered seriously either proposal, and the home care entitlement remains today open ended.

To be sure, the legislature did, in 1992, require the state Department of Social Services to develop a new system for assessing how many hours of home care individual clients are entitled to. The goal here was to minimize the extraordinary variation in hours among similarly situated clients (New York City clients, in particular, received far more home care hours than did similarly situated clients in other communities).[30] Once again, however, client advocates and home care agencies immediately challenged the assessment system developed by the state bureaucrats, and as of late 1994 the new system had yet to be implemented.

Increased Number of Clients

Beginning in the early 1980s, the number of clients receiving home care services rose dramatically. In New York City, for example, the caseload went from 17,000 in 1979 to over 29,000 in 1984.[31] The increased caseload clearly contributed to the dramatic rise in program expenditures. Personal care expenditures, for example, increased from $184 million in 1979 to $520 million in 1984.[32]

The increased caseload was due largely to the 1980 decision to privatize New York City's home attendant program. The newly hired social services agencies, unlike the public officials who previously supervised the program, actively publicized and promoted the home care options. These agencies had a mission of program expansion, and they had as well a blank check from Medicaid with which to pursue their goal. Not surprisingly, many Medicaid beneficiaries, previously unaware of the options available, signed up for service. The wave of new enrollments continued from 1980 until the mid-1980s.

Health Care Unions

During the early 1980s, unions representing New York City's nonprofessional health care workers enrolled large numbers of home attendants. Despite their union membership, however, these workers remained low paid, especially when compared to similarly situated workers in hospitals and nursing homes. To be sure, working conditions and benefits were better than they were pre-1980, before the attendants became employees of social services agencies. Nonetheless, by 1986, home attendants were paid, on average, only $4.15 per hour, just eighty cents above the minimum wage.[33]

In early 1987, the new leadership of Local 1199 of the Retail, Wholesale Department Store Union, which represented a large number of home attendants, began a campaign to increase wages and benefits. The union first convinced District Council 37 of the American Federation of State, City, and Municipal Employees (AFSCME) to join the cause and to form the "New York Labor Union Coalition for Home Care Workers." The Coalition then persuaded Manhattan Borough President David Dinkens to hold public hearings on the plight of home care workers. And the coalition scored a publicity coup when it persuaded the Reverend Jesse

Jackson and John Cardinal O'Connor (the leader of New York's Catholic community) to add their voices to the campaign. As one commentator noted:

> While the media led with headlines about the newsmaking get together of the politically conservative cardinal and the progressive reverend, the fact that the meeting was arranged by the unions and announced their endorsement of the [campaign] did not go unnoticed in City Hall or the governor's office. Later the same day, Jackson addressed a rally of about 6,000 home care workers and their supporters in front of City Hall. Just about every liberal and minority politician in the city jostled for space on the platform to reiterate his or her support for the workers.[34]

Over the next few months, the campaign escalated as the media wrote stories and editorials sympathetic to the workers. Finally, in March 1988, the unions, the home care agencies, the city, and the state agreed on a new contract: home attendants would receive $5.90 an hour and increased fringe benefits, for a total compensation increase of 42 percent.[35] It was an important union victory, and it provides home attendants with compensation close to (though still below) their counterparts in hospitals and nursing homes. But it also was an expensive settlement that contributes dramatically to rising home care expenditures.

The Advocacy Community

The advocacy community in New York is relatively powerful, particularly when compared to its counterparts around the country. The influence is generated, in part, by an active and aggressive legal services community that challenges in court most state and local efforts to restrict social welfare benefits. Oftentimes, the litigation prompts case settlement negotiations and bargaining over policy; sometimes public officials try to preempt litigation by beginning the bargaining process during the legislative or regulatory process. But advocacy influence is not the result of only adversarial relationships. Many state officials, for example, particularly those in social services bureaucracies, are former advocates themselves who share with the current advocates both goals and values. Moreover, New York's pluralistic and fragmented political environment offers advocates numerous opportunities to enter and influence the policy debate: the state and its local welfare districts, for example, have created numerous "policy advisory councils." And New York's political culture has long encouraged group participation and influence.

There are, as a result, several advocacy organizations that exercise important influence over home care policy. The State Communities Aid Association is particularly effective. These organizations have set as a high priority both establishing and preserving a liberally interpreted "right" to home care. For this reason, advocacy groups have led the opposition to proposals that would cap the number of hours home care beneficiaries can receive.

Many consumer advocates also oppose the state's effort to expand programs in which a small number of home attendants provide care for a large group of clients, all of whom reside in the same building or neighborhood. These programs, sometimes called "shared aide" or "cluster care" initiatives, are defended by Medicaid officials on both fiscal and programmatic grounds: they cost less money, and they arguably encourage beneficiaries to attend local senior citizen centers (or other similar agencies). According to many advocates, however, these programs illegally undermine the right to in-home medical services and could lead to a diminished quality of care.

To be sure, the state legislature, as part of its 1991 cost-containment initiative, required counties to consider if clients could be more efficiently served in a shared aide environment (or in a personal emergency response program in which clients stayed at home alone more often but had a walkie-talkie type device to allow immediate communication with emergency medical personnel). Nonetheless, advocate opposition to implementing these "efficiencies" has seriously slowed their implementation (for example, local officials know that the decision to limit a client's home care hours in exchange for a personal emergency walkie-talkie is likely to be challenged by client advocates). As a result, by late 1994 fewer than three thousand of the hundred thousand personal care clients participated in shared aide programs.

Decentralized Governmental Administration

The two state agencies responsible for administering Medicaid's home care programs have extraordinarily different administrative techniques. The Department of Social Services, which oversees the personal care program, delegates nearly all authority (from application procedures to provider certification to ratemaking) to the local social services districts. While the department occasionally reviews and audits local programs, its influence is limited. The Department of Health, in contrast, seeks to limit local variation in the state's home health care program, adopting in Albany the rules and rates for every certified home health care agency.

Given their contrasting styles, the two agencies rarely work together or coordinate program activities.[36] Despite this administrative distance, however, actions taken by one agency often affect the other. For example, the Department of Health neither participated in nor authorized the 1987 settlement with New York City home attendants. Nonetheless, Department of Health officials felt bound to offer a similar package to home health workers employed by its programs.[37]

Ultimately, however, Department of Health officials generally share the premise that home care is usually more cost effective and humane than is institutionalization. Indeed, by regulating closely the development of new nursing home beds, the department itself encourages the growing demand for in-home services. With state officials thus in accord on this guiding principal and with a policy environment dominated by home care agencies, client advocates, and health care unions, New York's home care system continues to be expansive and expensive.

Policy in California: An Ongoing Commitment to Cost Containment

Prior to 1993, California's system of home care resembled the system in place prior to 1973 in New York: Medicare paid for certified home health aides who provided primarily short-term medical services, while the public assistance system paid for home attendants who provided nonmedical supportive services to the chronically ill and disabled. But while New York enacted a Medicaid-funded personal care program more than twenty years ago, California resisted this option until recently. And while New York's Medicaid program spends billions on home care services, both Medi-Cal and California's public assistance program have kept home care expenditures relatively low.

The comparison of California's public assistance home care program (called the In-Home Supportive Services program, or IHSS) and New York's Medicaid-funded personal care program is especially dramatic: California's program serves twice as many people for less than half the cost. In fiscal year 1990/91, for example, the IHSS program provided home attendants for 151,000 persons at a cost of $641 million.[38] That same year, New York's personal care program provided aides to just under 75,000 clients at a cost of $1.4 billion.[39] The variation in Medicaid-funded home health expenditures is equally large. In fiscal year 1986/87, for example, Medi-Cal spent less than $9 million on traditional home health services,[40] while New York's program spent $131.3 million.[41]

California officials note with pride, however, that their fiscal commitment to home care is quite substantial, exceeding that of every state except New York. According to a survey of nine of the nation's larger states, not only did California rank second (after New York), its home care expenditures exceeded those of the next seven states combined.[42]

To accomplish this blend of commitment and constraint, California officials generally pay home attendants the minimum wage and provide few (if any) fringe benefits. Moreover, California's home attendants receive less training, have less supervision, and work far fewer hours than do their counterparts in New York. Why the interstate variation? Because interest groups that wield significant policymaking influence in New York (unions, advocates, and nonprofit social services agencies) exercise little influence in California.

Minimum Wages for a Nonunion Workforce

Most home attendants in California currently earn the minimum wage ($4.25 per hour).[43] Most receive few fringe benefits (and no health insurance, overtime pay, or annual leave). In New York City, in contrast, home attendants received, back in 1989, a compensation package (of wages and fringe benefits) valued at $8.83 per hour. Even rural New York home attendants received, in 1989, a compensation package valued at $6.05 per hour.[44]

The wage differentials explain much of the variation in cost between California's and New York's programs. For example, California officials estimate that every penny added to home attendant salaries adds $1 million to the program's annual cost.[45] Accepting this assumption, if California's home attendants earned salaries equal to their New York City counterparts, California's annual home care costs would increase by $458 million, to well over $1 billion.

In California, home attendants are neither organized nor influential. Indeed, 91 percent of the attendant workforce are "independent providers" hired directly by the client, while only 8 percent work for social services agencies, and 1 percent are county employees.[46] These independent providers have little contact with each other or with some common organization. Very few belong to a labor union. Many (over 50 percent) are relatives or long-time friends of their client. Nearly all are poor and female and members of a racial minority. Some are themselves on welfare, supplementing their cash assistance with part-time employment. All belong to a population that sorely lacks political clout.

There are, to be sure, ongoing efforts to organize California's home attendants. Both the Service Employees and Industrial Union (SEIU) and the United Domestic Workers Union are campaigning to unionize the independent-provider home attendants. By and large, however, neither union is succeeding. It is too hard to organize poor women who work for themselves in thousands of homes around the state. Indeed, even in New York City, with its history and tradition of powerful health care unions, home attendants were not successfully organized until they became employees of nonprofit social services agencies (in 1980). Earlier efforts to organize independent-provider home attendants had failed.

It is quite unlikely, moreover, that many California counties will abandon the independent contractor system and adopt instead a large-scale contract agency approach.[47] To the contrary, the trend today is toward increased reliance on the individual provider approach. According to state officials, for example, three counties recently abandoned the contract agency approach, substituting in its place an exclusive reliance on individual providers. County officials cited as persuasive the lower cost and increased flexibility of the individual provider approach. In contrast, only one county has in recent years hired for the first time a home attendant agency, and that county continues to rely upon numerous individual providers as well.[48]

Given this political environment, government officials determine home attendant reimbursement in an autonomous and centralized fashion. There is little need to consult or consider the interests of the workers themselves. There is, instead, a government-supported minimum-wage industry.

Little Training and Less Supervision

California's home attendants, unlike their New York counterparts, receive little (if any) training or supervision. Indeed, attendants (at least the 91 percent who are "independent providers") are considered employees of the beneficiaries, and it is the beneficiaries who train and supervise. The situation that results is often disastrous. Attendants work with needy and occasionally demanding clients, and do so without the guidance, support, or oversight of any public bureaucracy. The home attendants' job, stressful in the best of circumstances, often becomes unbearable. At the same time, however, client needs are often unmet by the unskilled, untrained, and oftentimes unmotivated workforce. Not surprisingly, client dissatisfaction is quite high.[49]

To be sure, some clients prosper under the informal system. Young disabled clients, for example, often appreciate the discretion they enjoy in shaping relationships with their attendants.[50] Similarly, clients who hire friends or family members as attendants sometimes prefer an uninvolved government bureaucracy. Moreover, some workers and clients overcome all obstacles and forge close and even loving relationships. Nonetheless, for large numbers of beneficiaries, the lack of worker training and the absence of governmental oversight is disturbing (and potentially dangerous).[51]

Despite its drawbacks, the laissez-faire system is likely to continue. County opposition to hiring home attendant agencies stems, in part, from the belief that the training these agencies provide their workers is simply too expensive. Program officials have clearly decided that it is preferable to provide many clients with untrained and poorly paid attendants than to provide fewer clients with better-trained and better-paid attendants.

Capping the Number of Home Care Hours

California's home attendant clients receive far fewer hours of care than do their counterparts in New York. In 1988, for example, the average IHSS client received 75.5 hours per month of home attendant care.[52] In New York, in contrast, the average client received over 200 hours of care per month.[53] Similarly, a "nonseverely impaired" California client can receive no more than 195 hours of care per month, while a "severely impaired" client is limited to 283 hours.[54] In New York, in contrast, 17 percent of home attendant clients receive care twenty-four hours per day, seven days a week (or over 700 hours of care per month).[55]

The variation in home attendant hours is explained best by the variation in state policymaking environments. In New York, the key nongovernmental players (home attendant agencies, social workers, union leaders, and client advocates) have nurtured the notion that beneficiaries are entitled to whatever home care services they might benefit from. Government officials, and the courts, have accepted this assumption. In California, in contrast, government officials strongly reject the proposition that home care is or ought to be an open-ended entitlement. And while California's system is in many respects quite fragmented (particularly with clients choosing their own attendants), state officials have shaped the culture that guides the program and the dollars that support it.

Maximizing Federal Revenue: The Decision to Implement a Personal Care Program

In April 1993, California implemented for the first time a Medi-Cal-funded personal care program. By all accounts, the new program is intended primarily to provide increased federal funding for the state's ongoing home attendant program (the IHSS program). The program was adopted, however, only after a long and vigorous debate over whether its enactment would reduce state control over home care policy, thereby reducing state cost-containment autonomy. State officials went along with the change only after convincing themselves that the additional federal dollars would not undermine state program control.

The fiscal argument in favor of a personal care program was straightforward. The IHSS program was funded by a combination of federal Title XX funds (which could be spent on a wide array of programs) and state and local funds. If all (or most) IHSS recipients were converted to personal care recipients, the state could spend the freed up Title XX funds (some $325 million) on other social services programs (such as day care) and still receive 50 percent federal funding for the new Medi-Cal service. The result would be a large infusion of federal dollars.

There was also a programmatic argument in favor of a personal care program: many IHSS recipients go without needed in-home medical services because their home attendants are neither qualified nor permitted to perform such tasks. Personal care attendants, however, are (theoretically) trained to perform a range of medical services and are supervised by registered nurses. Adopting a personal care program would thus enable clients to obtain needed services and to do so largely at federal expense.

To be sure, some in the advocacy community remained skeptical. Many disabled clients, for example, were concerned that a personal care program would reduce their ability to direct the activities of attendants. Other IHSS recipients (and workers) were troubled by a provision in federal Medicaid law that prohibits family members from acting as attendants.[56]

Ironically, however, the primary obstacle to a personal care program came not from these advocates, however, but from skeptical state officials who had for years challenged the argument that the new program would be cost free. The fiscal pessimism was rooted in several assumptions. First, since many IHSS services are (arguably) insufficiently "medical" to be transferred to a personal care program, the IHSS program would not disappear. Second, even if IHSS could be fully medicalized, it wouldn't be: seven-hundred-million-dollar programs rarely disappear. Third, medicalizing IHSS would itself raise costs. Attendants presumably would receive training and supervision, which is expensive. Attendants also would increasingly perform technologically sophisticated (and expensive) medical treatments.

For years, the state's fiscal pessimists (lodged in both the Department of Health Services and the Department of Finance), defeated every effort to adopt a personal care program. In 1992, however, the political environment shifted during the state's difficult budget crisis when state officials not only transferred an increased percentage of the IHSS cost to the counties, but also imposed (in September) an across-the-board 12.5 percent cutback in the hours of care received by every client.[57] County leaders, consumer advocates, and union officials (especially those in the Service Employees and Industrial Union) challenged the cutbacks, suggesting that adopting a personal care program could have avoided the crisis (because of the extra federal revenue). This time the administration agreed: the state adopted a personal care program and restored the service cutbacks.

The fiscal pessimists were not totally convinced. But several factors tipped the scale. First, newly elected Governor Pete Wilson, a former United States senator, was far more interested in maximizing federal revenues than were his predecessors. Second, the proposal promised to end the controversy engendered by the IHSS cutbacks, and to do so with primarily federal funds. Third, and perhaps most important, Medi-Cal officials were finally persuaded that adopting personal care did not mean losing programmatic (or fiscal) control, particularly since the individual provider system could remain in place and the cap on hours could remain as well.

California's Home Care Agencies: A For-Profit Industry Avoids Medi-Cal

In California, as in other states, home care refers both to the federally required home health care program (under which states reimburse nurses and other medical providers for care rendered to beneficiaries eligible for but not receiving nursing home care) and to the optional home attendant programs (such as the personal care program and the various state waiver programs). There is, however, little overlap in the workforce that provides care under the various programs. Most California home attendants work as independent contractors, are hired directly by clients, receive little training and supervision, are paid the minimum wage, and often are themselves on welfare. Home health care workers, in contrast, are professionally trained, generally work for one of the approximately four hundred for-profit home health agencies in the state,[58] are often unionized, and receive relatively good wages and benefits.

Rather remarkably, however, only about ten home health agencies participate routinely in Medi-Cal. The reason most often cited is low reimbursement. Most agencies prefer working with Medicare clients (or those with private insurance): the pay is better. In 1987, for example, Medicare reimbursed the average Los Angeles agency nearly $75 per visit; Medi-Cal paid less than $58 for the same care.[59]

Home health agencies also complain regularly about Medi-Cal laws and regulations that strictly limit client eligibility to home health services and impose bureaucratic hoops for clients and workers to hurdle. The state has, for example, an administratively burdensome prior authorization procedure. The state also imposes an overall cap on the number of authorized visits available to any client. As a result, Medi-Cal beneficiaries receive far fewer home health visits than do similarly situated beneficiaries in other states. In 1987, for example, Medi-Cal-funded home health workers visited an average client 7 times a year, as compared with 140 visits by a typical New York worker, 19 visits by a Pennsylvania worker, and 15 visits by an Illinois worker.[60]

The state-imposed barriers to home health care, along with the low provider participation, enable state officials to control tightly the funds expended on Medi-Cal home health care services. The contrast with New York could hardly be sharper. In that state, nonprofit social services agencies, working with consumer advocates, union leaders, and sympathetic state and local officials, have created an expensive and expansive home health care program. As I noted earlier, in fiscal year 1986/87, New York's Medicaid home health expenditures totalled $131.3 million; California's program that same year spent around $9 million. Here, as in the home attendant programs described previously, the state's dissimilar policymaking environments have produced vastly dissimilar policy outcomes.

7

Reducing the Cost of Hospital Care: Lessons from New York and California

Hospitals and the Poor

The primary mission of the United States' first hospitals, which were formed during the eighteenth century, was to provide medical care to poor people. Most of these hospitals were publicly owned. New York City's Bellevue Hospital, for example, began as an infirmary to New York's Almshouse for the poor.[1] Others were privately operated "charity" institutions, such as the Massachusetts General Hospital. All were avoided by the middle class, who complained (legitimately) about overcrowded wards and poor hygienic conditions, and who received care instead from private physicians making house calls.

During the late nineteenth century, however, four developments prompted dramatic growth in both the size and status of the hospital industry. First, advances in medical technology (such as the inventions of antiseptics, anesthesia, and x-rays) encouraged wealthier patients to utilize hospitals, thereby eliminating much of the prior social stigma. Second, the number of nurses expanded dramatically, and hospital-based nurses worked hard to improve hygienic conditions. Third, the growing urbanization and industrialization of American life produced an increasingly rootless society, which, in turn, lessened the ability of families to care for their

sick at home. Fourth, and finally, doctors were becoming less willing to make house calls, preferring instead the efficiencies of scale
now provided in a hospital.[2]

For all of these reasons, the nation's hospital stock grew from
less than two hundred in 1873 to nearly seven thousand by 1930.[3]
Then, after World War II, Congress itself encouraged another dramatic expansion in the nation's hospital bed supply when it enacted the Hill-Burton program, which provided federal funds to
stimulate hospital construction and modernization.[4] The policy
assumption was that all Americans should have access to the increasingly sophisticated medical care rendered in state-of-the-art
hospital facilities. By the mid-1970s, Hill-Burton had generated
another 400,000 hospital beds, many in rural communities.

As the hospital industry grew, however, hospitals themselves
were increasingly providing dual-track care: persons with money
(or insurance) were treated in private rooms by private physicians;
persons unable to pay were treated in large open wards by hospital
staff (or medical students). This was true both in public hospitals
(which treated a predominately indigent population) and in the
more prestigious private facilities (even when the local welfare
department partially subsidized the cost of care).

To be sure, the enactment of Medicaid was expected to lead to a
decline in the dual-track system. Hospitals would receive the same
cost-based reimbursement from Medicaid that they received from
Medicare and private insurers. Public and private hospitals would
compete for the Medicaid client. Poor people would receive mainstream care. Unfortunately, however, the reformers' vision of medical equality was never realized. Part of the problem was the unexpected and unprecedented rise in hospital costs, which began in
the late 1960s, and was attributable largely to the cost-based reimbursement required by both the Medicare and Medicaid statutes.
As Eli Ginzberg notes,

> Hospitals suddenly were in an environment in which the
> more they spent, the better. There was no point to their

continuing to pursue fiscally conservative policies. In fact, they ran the risk of losing out to competitors unless they acquired the most recent equipment, often before its efficacy had been fully established; unless they added more professional and support staff to increase the flow of patients they could treat; unless they raised salaries and fringe benefits and thus attracted and retained better professional and support staffs.[5]

In this changed environment, states shifted their policy emphasis from mainstreaming the poor to reducing and containing hospital costs. These efforts typically focused on Medicaid, though some states adopted a more global approach. The politics of hospital reimbursement were soon difficult, explosive, and complicated.

New York: The Pre-Medicaid Era

New York City has long provided expansive hospital services to its poor. In 1794, for example, the city established Bellevue, one of the nation's first public hospitals. The city later created several other public facilities and, by the early twentieth century, had the nation's largest municipal hospital system. Moreover, by the 1930s, the city was also reimbursing private hospitals for care rendered to welfare recipients.[6] But the city (like other New York communities) controlled the level of its generosity with little interference from the state or federal governments. For example, while the state's Department of Social Services would suggest rates to be paid to private hospitals, the final decision was up to local welfare commissioners, and that decision depended more on local budget calculations than on recommendations from state officials.[7]

The era of local control ended, however, in early 1966, when the state legislature enacted Article 28 of the state's Public Health Law and the federal government enacted the Medicare and Medicaid programs. The new state law, enacted by an activist and liberal state legislature, required the state to fund 50 percent of the cost of hospital care provided to the poor. The policy assumption was that state funds would encourage local governments (especially those outside of New York City) to provide additional services. At the same time, however, the law required the state's commissioner of health to both establish the actual rates to be paid and ensure that such rates were reasonably related to the costs incurred by the hospitals.[8] No longer would rates be negotiated between county officials and hospital administrators. Instead, under the reimbursement methodology developed by the state commissioner, state officials would use a hospital's costs from two years before, adjusted for inflation, to develop a daily rate for each welfare client. Hospitals' charges thereafter for the welfare population would be easily calculated: the daily rate times the number of clients.

Ironically, however, just as the state was implementing its changed reimbursement system, the newly enacted Medicaid program was requiring a very different approach. Under the new federal regime, state Medicaid programs were to reimburse hospitals retroactively for their actual costs, regardless of whether such costs were above or below some preset daily rate. Since federal officials were unwilling to exempt New York from the federal requirements, the state (reluctantly) abandoned its newly developed per diem system.

Policy in New York, 1966–1969:
The Movement toward Rate Regulation

By 1967, Medicaid, Medicare, and most private insurers were all reimbursing hospitals retroactively for their actual costs. This methodology was extraordinarily inflationary: the higher the hospitals' costs, the higher its reimbursement. The system was also inequitable as it rewarded costs not quality (or efficiency). Historians Robert Stevens and Rosemary Stevens describe what happened next: "some small hospitals discovered that, faced with a disorganized bureaucracy, they could recover from Medicaid anything they spent. Thus, some small hospitals were being paid more than $90 per day, while Columbia-Presbyterian Medical Center received only $76.95 for ward care, despite its highly specialized staff and facilities."[9]

Despite the rise in costs, hospitals around the country were generally successful in resisting state cost-containment efforts. Not only were hospitals influential political actors, but the payer community (both insurers and government) was generally fragmented and weak. In New York, however, state officials, still itching to try the shelved per diem reimbursement methodology, had an important ally, the nation's largest and most powerful Blue Cross plan. Blue Cross officials, unusually independent from the local hospital industry and anxious to reduce their hospital care payments, proposed early in 1969 a thirty-three month freeze on hospital rates charged to Blue Cross and Medicaid. While the proposal would, if enacted, surely violate federal Medicaid law, which required that hospitals be reimbursed by Medicaid for their "reasonable costs" (costs that clearly would not stay frozen for nearly three years), the hardball tactics worked: under a compromise arrangement the freeze was reduced to nine months,[10] the state developed prospective Medicaid and Blue Cross rates (to be implemented after the freeze) that were "reasonably related to the costs of efficient production of [hospital] services,"[11] and the federal government (by now itself concerned about rising hospital costs) permitted New York's "demonstration project" to proceed.[12]

Policy in New York, 1969–1975: Rate Regulation Produces Disappointing Results

New York's new reimbursement system did not produce the significant savings that were expected. Instead, the early 1970s saw a continual rise in hospital costs. Why the higher costs? Three explanations seem persuasive. First, the Health Department regulations implementing the legislation were unexpectedly generous to the hospital industry. Second, the state's powerful health care unions obtained generous wage settlements. And third, patients in

New York's hospitals had unusually long (and thus expensive) hospital stays.

Regulatory Givebacks

The new system required the state's Department of Health to examine a hospital's costs from two years before, adjust them for inflation, compare them with costs incurred by similarly situated hospitals, disallow them to the extent they were 10 percent higher than those of their counterparts, and use the results to develop a daily reimbursement rate. By regulatory fiat, however, the department exempted from the new system "capital costs, costs of schools of nursing, costs of interns and residents, and costs of ancillary services."[13] These exemptions were enormously helpful to the high-cost (and politically powerful) teaching hospitals, which could still receive full reimbursement for the actual costs of the exempted items and also shift routine costs to ancillary budgets and thereby inflate their budgets even further.[14]

A second loophole, also a plum for the academic medical centers, was the decision to classify hospitals by type and sponsorship (as well as by size and location). As a result, high-cost academic institutions were compared with their academic competitors, and both could invest in the latest medical technology, perform the most expensive medical procedures, and utilize the most inefficient administrative techniques.

Finally, the department built into the ratemaking process an elaborate appeals procedure, enabling hospitals to seek rate revisions to cover expansions of services, improvements in patient care, and other assorted expenditures. Hospitals used the appeals procedure to obtain rate increases well beyond those initially approved.

Generous Wage Settlements

During the early 1960s, union organizers began a campaign to represent New York City's nonprofessional hospital workforce.[15] Hospital workers at that time endured low wages, poor working conditions, and high turnover. Within a few years, however, most hospital workers were union members, wages and benefits were dramatically increased, and labor costs were inflating Medicaid expenditures.

The union victories were due, in large part, to the coalition between union leaders and civil rights advocates. After all, the civil rights movement was turning away from the south and toward the urban north, hospitals were the primary employer of urban blacks, and economic justice was becoming the movement's new demand. The alliance was politically powerful because workers enrolled in unions in unprecedented numbers (encouraged by a nonprofit and public hospital system that was surprisingly receptive) and because city and state officials concluded that union victories produced political benefits. New York City Mayor John Lindsay and Governor Nelson Rockefeller were especially anxious to mollify labor leaders.[16]

The pro-labor environment soon produced generous wage settlements: 24 percent in 1966, 25 percent in 1968, and similar increases during the early 1970s.[17] Moreover, state officials built these increases into the Medicaid and Blue Cross rates by developing a concept (also used in nursing home reimbursement) called the "substitute labor price movement" (or "slip-ems"), pursuant to which negotiated wage increases were substituted for inflation-based increases, and hospital Medicaid reimbursement rates were increased accordingly.

The Long Lengths of Stay of New York's Hospital Patients

New Yorkers tend to have unusually long inpatient hospital stays. In 1987, for example, the average length of stay for a New York Medicaid patient was 11.3 days; the average stay for a Medi-Cal patient in California was only 6.3 days.[18] One explanation for the length-of-stay statistics is demographics. New York City, for example, has an unusually old, sick, uneducated, and rootless population.[19]

The composition of New York's medical infrastructure is a second factor. New York has many large teaching hospitals (over 15 percent of the nation's doctors are trained in New York), and doctors in teaching facilities generally perform high numbers of tests and procedures (both because they have the most sophisticated medical equipment and because testing is done for teaching as well as diagnostic purposes). New York also is home to more nonteaching facilities than are comparable cities (such as Los Angeles), and health researchers have long suggested that excess beds lead to excess utilization.[20]

The rate regulation system put in place in 1969 is, however, a third factor contributing to the state's long length of stay numbers. In a flat-rate reimbursement system, such as that then employed in New York, hospitals have a financial incentive to increase patients' lengths of stay, particularly since the first few days of hospitalization when the patient is diagnosed and stabilized are the most expensive, while later hospital days become far cheaper (often well below the daily reimbursement level).[21] For this reason, the longer the length of stay, the greater the hospital profit.

Policy in New York, 1975–1977: A Budget Crisis Produces Cost Containment

By mid-1975, both New York City and New York State were in the midst of fiscal crises. For nearly two years, the crises prompted a radical departure from the pluralistic policymaking that had long dominated hospital policymaking in New York. Key decisions were made by a handful of cost-conscious legislative staffers with little input from Medicaid officials, hospital lobbyists, or union leaders. As a result, Medicaid spending on hospitals declined significantly. By 1978, however, the tide shifted away from autonomous decision making and cost containment, and hospital politics was again a pluralistic policy arena.

The cost-containment era began on January 1, 1976, when the state legislature froze 1976 hospital inpatient rates at 1975 levels and legislative leaders directed a handful of staffers to develop a new and more stringent reimbursement methodology. This pol-

icymaking autonomy was particularly apparent in 1976 when the
staffers drafted most of the cost-containment bill in a single weekend session, and the hospital industry complained that it had been
sandbagged. In 1977, these same staffers engineered a second and
even more stringent cost-containment initiative, this time despite
the vehement opposition of the hospitals.

The cost-containment bills contained a three-pronged strategy.
First, they closed several loopholes in the rate-setting methodology in an effort to reduce the per diem rates paid to hospitals.
Second, they required increased utilization review to ensure that
persons receiving hospital care actually needed hospital care. And
third, they encouraged agency efforts to strictly enforce certificate-
of-need laws and to institute a program to close "unnecessary"
hospitals.

Closing the Loopholes

The cost-containment legislation tightened the reimbursement
methodology in five important respects. First, it declared that ancillary costs (on items such as x-rays and drugs) would be subject
to the same cost ceilings as other costs (previously ancillary costs
were reimbursed in full). Second, it reduced the ceiling on permissible costs from 110 percent of those incurred by similarly situated
hospitals to 100 percent. Otherwise put, hospital costs that exceeded the average costs of comparable hospitals would not be
reimbursed. Third, the inflation-trend factor (or the cost-of-living
increase hospitals received) was reduced significantly. Fourth, the
legislation penalized hospitals that failed to meet minimum occupancy levels (thereby encouraging hospitals to decertify underutilized beds). Fifth, and finally, the legislation penalized hospitals
that had patient lengths of stay longer than average (thereby encouraging hospitals to discharge patients more promptly).

Utilization Review

The cost-containment legislation initiated a program in which
state-funded nurses reviewed the care of Medicaid clients in sixty of

the state's largest hospitals, uncovering and discouraging unnecessary or excessive treatment. Medicaid then refused to reimburse any care determined to be unnecessary. Not surprisingly, these nurses were distrusted and disliked by most hospital staff, especially the doctors, who were unused to second guessing, especially by nurses. While the program never operated smoothly, and while physicians were often able to appeal and overturn treatment denials, the nurses had an admitted chilling effect on treatment decisions and thereby generated significant cost savings.

Closing Hospitals

In an effort to illustrate its commitment to cost containment, the legislature elevated to cabinet-level status the director of the Office of Health Systems Management, the unit within the state Health Department responsible both for developing reimbursement rates and enforcing certificate-of-need requirements. With his power base secured, the newly appointed director, Richard Berman, began a campaign to reduce the state's supply of hospital beds. First, Berman's staffers enforced strictly the state's certificate-of-need requirements, denying numerous requests for hospital construction or expansion. More dramatically, however, Berman instituted a program to close "unnecessary" hospitals throughout the state.

The closure campaign targeted hospitals that had both low occupancy levels and a record of poor patient care. The campaign quickly identified several large New York City hospitals, each located in a poverty-stricken community, as candidates for closure. Not surprisingly, the campaign generated significant opposition as consumer advocates complained about reduced access, union leaders worried about lost jobs, and civil rights activists alleged discrimination. Despite the opposition, however, twelve New York City hospitals, with approximately 4,500 beds (or 11 percent of the city's total bed population) were closed between 1975 and 1979.[22]

Policy in New York, 1978 to the Present: Pluralism Returns and Remains

By the late 1970s, with revenues from Medicaid (and Blue Cross) declining, the financial condition of New York's hospitals began to deteriorate. The state's private institutions, for example, were soon losing over 3 percent annually, at a time when hospitals around the country continued to make money.[23] In an effort to stem the fiscal bleeding, the hospital industry challenged in court nearly every aspect of the state's cost-containment initiative. Time and again, however, the courts sided with the state.

In *New York City Health and Hospitals Corp. v. Blum* (708 F. 2d 880 [2d Cir. 1983]), for example, the court rejected a challenge to the length-of-stay disallowance in the new reimbursement methodology. Similarly, in *Hospital Association of New York State v. Toia* (577 F. 2d 790 [2d Cir. 1978]), the court, while agreeing that the state's temporary freeze on hospital rates was illegal, rejected the hospitals' claim for retroactive monetary relief, declaring that the doctrine of sovereign immunity shielded the state from any such claims. And on several occasions, courts upheld the state's right to close or scale back underutilized facilities (or departments within larger institutions).

The hospital industry next tried to recoup lost revenue by shifting costs to the unregulated commercial health insurers and by cancelling affiliations with Blue Cross plans. The effort to shift costs increased the tension between the commercial insurers, hospitals, and Blue Cross. Ironically, however, it also created an alliance among the three groups: all were united in an effort to challenge the state's hospital reimbursement scheme. By mid-1977, the alliance included also the health care unions (which had done very poorly in their 1976 negotiations), New York City officials (who were spending more and more city dollars in an effort to keep public hospitals afloat), health care advocates (who noted the precarious fiscal condition of hospitals that served the poor), and civil rights leaders (concerned about lost jobs for a minority-dominated nonprofessional workforce).

The antistate coalition, powerful in its own right, was aided also by the end of the state's fiscal crisis (which undermined the perceived need for a strong and centralized cost-containment effort) and by Governor Hugh Carey's need for the coalition's political support during his 1978 reelection campaign.

In this context, Governor Carey devised a strategy to provide short-term help for those groups adversely affected by the cost-containment measures (to regain their political support) and to simultaneously develop a new institutional mechanism for making hospital reimbursement policy (to assuage those budget watchdogs who feared a return to long-term inflation).

The changed environment was evident, for example, during the 1978 negotiations between the voluntary hospitals and Local 1199. The union wanted a significant wage increase to make up for its poor showing in 1976. The hospitals were unwilling to finance an increase, citing fiscal losses imposed by the cost-containment package. A bitter strike seemed likely. Governor Carey, however, intervened on behalf of the union, and the three-way negotiations resulted in a 14.5 percent wage increase funded by increased Medicaid and Blue Cross rates[24] (available only because the state revived the so-called slip-em procedure, whereby negotiated wage increases are substituted for inflation-based increases).

The state also relaxed some of the more restrictive elements of the cost-containment package (such as the requirement that hospital costs that exceed those of similarly situated facilities be disallowed), thereby providing hospitals with more money. At the same time, however, the state provided short-term relief to the commercial insurance industry (by regulating, for the first time, the rates hospitals charged such insurers). And while Blue Cross officials were unhappy with rate increases, they were at least able to persuade several hospitals to renew their Blue Cross contracts (as the rate differential between Blue Cross and the commercial plans lessened).

In addition to these short-term measures, however, the governor and the legislature agreed to delegate the task of revising and overseeing the hospital reimbursement system to a new pluralistic agency, called the Council on Health Care Financing, that was composed of members of the legislature, the hospitals, Blue Cross, the commercial insurers, the unions, and the advocates. By including the key interest groups in the new governing body, the state confirmed the changed nature of the hospital policymaking arena. The single-minded quest to control costs, which dominated during the fiscal crisis, was replaced by pluralistic bargaining, aimed at reviving the hospital industry, stabilizing the insurance industry, and maintaining a regulatory cost-containment approach.

Early on, the council developed a consensus on two goals: first, a single-payment methodology for all payers (which would minimize cost shifting and provide a more stable reimbursement environment); and second, a surcharge on hospital revenue with the funds collected to be used to subsidize hospitals for a portion of their uncompensated care and to offer financial support for hospitals in fiscal distress.[25]

There was, to be sure, lengthy debate over the mechanics of the new system, particularly with respect to the formula by which the bad debt and charity pool would be distributed. Eventually, however, the council reached agreement on the specifics of a proposal (which shifted most of the bad-debt money to upstate private hospitals on the theory that the city itself subsidizes the bad debt of its own hospitals). Shortly thereafter, the state received permission from the federal government to calculate Medicare rates in New York using the same prospective per diem methodology used to calculate Medicaid, Blue Cross, and all other hospital rates. Then, in January 1983, the New York Prospective Hospital Reimbursement Methodology (NYPHRM) went into effect.

Within months, the financial condition of the state's hospitals had improved significantly. After losing nearly $90 million in 1982, the state's voluntary and proprietary hospitals produced a net profit of nearly $19 million in 1983.[26] Indeed, while analysts often argue (with merit) that all-payer reimbursement systems reduce costs,[27] the all-payer system in New York represented a dramatic (and perhaps warranted) retreat from a truly effective cost-containment experiment.

To be sure, the new system did lessen the amount of Medicare revenue generated by most hospitals since the state reimbursement levels were below the unusually high Medicare rates. But Medicare was then developing its own cost-containment program, under which a hospital's reimbursement would depend largely on the patient's diagnosis, and many hospitals preferred the security of New York's regulated system to the insecurity of a federal cost-containment regime. As the new federal system evolved, however, many hospitals regretted their decision. The state's teaching hospitals were particularly upset to discover that the new federal system provided teaching hospitals (everywhere but New York) with a significant bonus to compensate for the higher costs incurred in educating doctors.[28] These hospitals now wanted Medicare patients to be reimbursed by the federal government, under the new federal system, and not by the state, under the state's all-payer system. The Council on Health Care Financing was agreeable, and, as of 1986, Medicare was no longer included in the state-regulated system. The result was a $686.2 million fiscal windfall for the state's teaching hospitals.[29]

By 1987, however, with hospital revenue rising, the council grew increasingly divided. There was now tension between the state's commissioner of health, David Axelrod, and much of the state's hospital industry. Three issues dominated the debate. First, Axelrod distrusted the hospitals' ongoing claims of fiscal crisis. Second, Axelrod was anxious to restructure the state's system of medical education, encouraging the production of fewer medical specialists and more primary care physicians. And third, Axelrod sought to regulate the day-to-day activities of New York's hospitals to an unprecedented degree. The era of goodwill and consensual politics was over. Moreover, since NYPHRM needs to be renewed every two to three years, the pluralistic battling rarely abates.

In 1988, for example, the Health Department and the industry battled fiercely over the proposal that the state adopt a case-payment system to replace the per diem rates then paid by Medicaid, Blue Cross, and the other state-regulated payers. The Department of Health recommended that reimbursement in the new system depend almost entirely on the patient's diagnosis. The hospitals, fearing a sharp decline in revenue, suggested that reimbursement remain primarily dependent on actual costs, but with a minor adjustment to reflect the patient's diagnosis. The council and then the legislature sided with the hospitals, adopting a case-payment system favorable to the industry. Governor Mario Cuomo, following Axelrod's advice, vetoed the measure. The parties then compromised, enacting a bill that split the difference between the hospitals and the Health Department.

Two years later, in 1990, the skirmishing grew more intense. The hospitals claimed that 70 percent of the state's hospitals were losing money and the industry as a whole was losing billions.[30] The Health Department challenged the hospitals' figures as wildly exaggerated and noted also that most of the losses were borne by public hospitals (which received local subsidies to cover their losses), and that the losses were almost all on outpatient care (thereby suggesting that the case-payment inpatient rates were adequate).[31] The department then recommended that any increased reimbursement be limited to outpatient care, both to target funds where they were needed most and to simultaneously expand the primary care infrastructure. Once again, however, the council and then the legislature sided with the industry, enacting a bill that not only provided the industry with a 14 percent reimbursement increase (or around $420 million), but also targeted nearly all of the increase (around $380 million) for inpatient care (primarily for higher nursing salaries).

As in 1988, the Health Department urged the governor to veto the bill. This time, however, Cuomo rejected his agency's advice. One factor in his decision was the inclusion in the bill of $20 million to begin a state-subsidized health insurance plan for working-class children. Cuomo (and many health care advocates) envisioned this program as a first step toward universal health insurance, and legislative Republicans warned that the program would be tabled indefinitely if not enacted then. Cuomo was also concerned about the political influence of the hospitals. As the *New York Times* reported: "legislative and administration officials had speculated that Mr. Cuomo would not veto the bill in an election year, when he then would have to tell voters why he opposed a bill that bailed out hospitals in every corner of the state and provided health insurance for poor children."[32]

With reimbursement disputes growing increasingly partisan, the council became increasingly irrelevant. Legislative and executive leaders, hospital lobbyists, and other interest-group players (including the unions, the insurers, and the business community) took their positions public, eschewing the behind-the-scenes consensus building that dominated the council's early efforts. Nevertheless, by 1993, the intramural battling over hospital reimbursement had become predictable. The hospitals pleaded poverty. The Health Department challenged the industry's numbers and pressed to target any reimbursement increases at outpatient and primary care. The legislature (especially the Republican-dominated state senate) sided with the industry and enacted a generous inpatient reimbursement increase (in 1993, the increase was $181 million, at a time when the department proposed actually reducing inpatient reimbursement). The governor signed the bill, both because of the hospitals' political clout and because the bill contained various incremental efforts to encourage more primary care practitioners. The parties then immediately geared up for the next legislative battle, two years hence.

Policy in California, 1966–1981: Federal Bureaucrats and the Courts Dominate the Policymaking Process

In 1982, the California legislature enacted the "selective contracting" program, pursuant to which hospitals bid for the right to treat Medi-Cal clients. This program, which has dramatically lowered the state's Medi-Cal hospital bill, is often touted as evidence that free-market competition can reduce health care costs. But selective contracting reduces costs not because California's big hospitals compete vigorously for Medi-Cal business but because powerful and autonomous state officials dictate to these hospitals the price they can charge for the Medi-Cal client. The California experience thus supports the thesis that centralized regulatory control leads to cost containment; it is not, as some suggest, an exception to the rule. Indeed, Medi-Cal officials spent the fifteen years prior to selective contracting trying unsuccessfully to snare the centralized authority they now enjoy.

The story begins with the federal command, in the original Medicaid statute, that state's reimburse hospitals for the actual cost of care rendered to beneficiaries. In California, as elsewhere, this methodology encouraged a rapid rise in hospital reimbursement. By the late 1960s, Medi-Cal officials, again like their counterparts elsewhere, were experimenting with various efforts to lower the state's inpatient hospital bill. The administrators adopted a three-pronged approach: first, institute strict utilization review procedures; second, transfer costs to county governments; and third, seek federal permission (much like New York) to move away from reasonable-cost reimbursement, substituting in its stead a state-established cap on expenditures.

Utilization Review

Medi-Cal administrators have long imposed unusually strict utilization review requirements: unable to control what hospitals charge (given the federal law governing hospital reimbursement), state officials could at least restrict how much care was rendered. Beginning in 1967, for example, the state required beneficiaries to obtain prior authorization for hospital stays of more than eight days in noncounty facilities. Three years later, Medi-Cal required prior authorization for all nonemergency hospitalizations—in all hospitals. Even emergency admissions were subject to strict utilization review; by 1975 emergency admissions without prior authorization were limited to three days, and by 1981 prior authorization was required for nearly all admissions (weekend admissions could be authorized on the following Monday).[33] While such Medicaid prior-authorization rules are today common, they were quite rare at the time.

According to at least one study, the prior-authorization requirements reduced beneficiary medical care utilization. The study demonstrated that in 1981, 28 percent of all requests to extend hospital stays were denied.[34] Three years earlier, treatment-authorization denials purportedly saved Medi-Cal over $16 million.[35] Some Medi-Cal officials claim the savings were even greater. Even Medi-Cal administrators acknowledge, however, that the savings were too low to significantly constrain rising costs. Other strategies were needed.

Shifting the Cost

The state-county dispute was rooted in the state's decision, in 1966, to develop the so-called county option program, under which counties paid a small percentage of the overall Medi-Cal bill, but the state guaranteed that county medical expenditures (for Medi-Cal beneficiaries and others) would not exceed (in real dollars) what the counties spent in 1964.

The county option program was an obvious target for cost-cutting state officials (like Ronald Reagan). As a savvy politician, however, Governor Reagan knew better than to eliminate the program without (purportedly) giving the counties something in return. He knew also that the county hospital system was struggling to care for large numbers of uninsured adults who were ineligible for Medi-Cal only because they weren't aged, blind, or disabled. The result was a 1971 law that eliminated the county option program and increased the county share of the Medi-Cal bill, but provided Medi-Cal eligibility to the so-called medically indigent adult (or "MIA") population. Reagan predicted that 800,000 persons would become Medi-Cal eligible, such adults could be cared for in the state's growing for-profit health care industry, and that the overall indigent care costs paid by the counties would go down. In Reagan's words: "In the development of every facet of this program, I have insisted that these reforms cause no net shift in costs to the already overburdened counties. I am confident that this will not happen and that most counties will be able to effect actual savings if the entire program is adopted."[36]

Despite Reagan's prediction, the 1971 legislation was a disaster for the counties. First, only about 250,000 indigent adults joined the Medi-Cal program, leaving the counties still responsible for almost 600,000 others. Now, however, there wasn't any state aid to help defray the cost. Second, the county share of the overall Medi-Cal bill rose dramatically, from $215 million in fiscal year 1970/71 to more than $410 million in fiscal year 1977/78.[37] To pay for their rising health bill, most counties increased local property taxes. In fiscal year 1971/72, counties collected $1.9 billion in property taxes, spending 22.7 percent of those funds on indigent health care. By 1977/78, the counties were collecting $2.8 billion and spending 35.5 percent on indigent care.[38]

By 1978, Reagan's "new federalism" approach (shift the burden to the counties) contributed to the California tax revolt of 1978, otherwise known as Proposition 13, which rolled back property tax levels and limited future tax increases.[39] With counties now unable to pay the health care bill, the state reluctantly assumed the county share of the Medi-Cal bill and even created a County Health Services Fund to ensure the continuation of minimal levels of county health services. The pendulum had shifted: now it was the state that was burdened with rising health care costs. Moreover, the state's ability to pay the health care bill was growing problematic: a severe recession, coupled with the cost of the county bailout and a decline in federal aid (under now President Ronald Reagan), placed the state in a precarious financial position. Indeed, a state budget surplus of $3.7 billion in 1978 was gone by 1982.[40]

Regulating Rates

In 1975, Medi-Cal administrators proposed a fixed annual cap on hospital reimbursement increases. Such a system would provide state officials with the same control over hospital rates that they had successfully wielded over nursing home rates. Federal officials approved the plan in March 1976. Before it could be implemented, however, a federal judge (in 1979) voided the plan on the grounds that the federal officials had not ensured that hospitals would be adequately reimbursed.[41]

Following the court's decision, Medi-Cal officials developed a revised rate regulation initiative. The new plan abandoned the effort to impose an overall fiscal cap, substituting in its stead caps on particular items (such as wages) but allowing open-ended increases for other items (such as depreciation). Before this plan was implemented, however, Congress (by passing the Boren Amendment) increased state discretion in developing hospital reimbursement systems. State officials took the federal action as a cue to try again their more restrictive cap on overall hospital reimbursement increases. Once again, however, the federal courts voided the plan, holding that "[s]tate DHS' adoption of the 6 percent cap without making a finding as to the reasonableness and adequacy of the proposed rates to meet the costs of efficiently and economically operated hospitals after considering all the relevant factors is arbitrary and inconsistent with law."[42]

Ironically, however, two days before the court's decision, on June 21, 1982, the California legislature had itself rejected the rate regulation approach, opting instead to enact the selective contracting system.

Policy in California, 1982 to the Present: State Bureaucrats Control Costs

The selective contracting program was first proposed, in 1978, by state senator John Garamendi.[43] While the program was not enacted that year, the concept grew increasingly attractive to cost-conscious Medi-Cal officials: why not have hospitals compete for Medi-Cal business? With occupancy levels in California's hospitals quite low,[44] and with many hospitals dependent on Medi-Cal revenue, state officials would be in a strong bargaining position.

The hospital industry was divided over the proposal. Many small for-profit facilities were attracted to the idea: it would enable them to opt out of the Medi-Cal program (except for services provided in the emergency room) and concentrate instead on their privately insured patient base. But the larger hospitals, especially those with large numbers of Medi-Cal patients, were vehemently opposed to selective contracting: it would delegate far too much authority to autonomous state administrators. These hospitals organized a determined effort to defeat the proposal. In May 1992, for example, approximately two hundred hospital officials rallied against the proposal on the steps of the capitol.[45] At the same time, the California Hospital Association began a major lobbying effort to defeat the proposal. In contrast to New York politics, however, the hospitals had very little ability to influence the policymaking debate. Three factors seem most important. First, many policymakers believed that hospitals (unlike nursing homes) had done quite well under Medi-Cal, largely because the state's efforts to regulate rates had consistently been rebuffed. This was an opportunity to balance the cost-containment burden. Second, selective contracting as a policy model had significant political appeal: the model promised savings induced by competition and was therefore far more attractive (to California policymakers) than the regulatory rate-setting (which the courts were rejecting anyway). Finally, the hospital industry was itself divided (with the small for-profits favoring the bill), thereby diluting the strength of the opposition. For all of these reasons, the selective contracting legislation was enacted into law in June 1982.

The new initiative was heralded as a path-breaking effort to introduce competition into the hospital industry. State officials would estimate the number of hospital beds needed for Medi-Cal patients; hospitals would bid for Medi-Cal contracts; hospitals without contracts would provide only emergency room care to Medi-Cal patients (for which they would receive cost-based reimbursement); and the competition for business would encourage efficiency and savings.

Selective contracting as implemented, however, was hardly a case study in competition. Instead, and to the contrary, selective contracting provided a backdoor route for powerful state officials to set (and thereby lower) reimbursement rates. The most powerful such official was William Guy, the so-called czar of the hospital contracting system. Guy's mission was to negotiate the first round of contracts; after that, the California Medical Assistance Commission (CMAC) would take over.

Guy was in a powerful bargaining position: most of California's large hospitals needed Medi-Cal contracts (particularly given their low occupancy rates). Using this leverage, Guy decided to implement a policy of "no net increases" in overall hospital expenditures, an even tougher fiscal cap than had previously been rejected by the federal courts. Such a policy was enormously distressing to hospitals used to double-digit cost-of-living increases. But Guy was unwilling to retreat. And in November 1982, he rejected bids proffered by San Francisco's three largest hospitals, hospitals that serviced 40 percent of San Francisco's Medi-Cal population. News of the rejection traveled quickly. In the words of one commentator:

> Exclusion of these hospitals sent a message to hospitals in the rest of the state that the state did not so highly value participation (and access for recipients) that it would accept bids that were not competitively priced. The state clearly had chosen to exercise much of the market power it had, and the hospitals now understood that fact. In the days following the San Francisco outcome, the state was flooded with phone calls from hospitals in other areas reducing their bids. The San Francisco area bidding process was reopened, and — this time — the three excluded hospitals submitted acceptable rates.[46]

By June 1983, 245 of the state's 526 general acute care hospitals had Medi-Cal contracts,[47] and most contracting hospitals accepted rates well below prior levels. Another 120 hospitals tried but failed to win contracts. The first year alone the program saved over $184 million in Medi-Cal expenditures.

In July 1983, CMAC assumed the task of administering the selective contracting program: it adopted and implemented the hard-nosed negotiating model developed by Bill Guy. Moreover, local politicians have generally been precluded from influencing the negotiating process: CMAC is an independent and autonomous institution that enjoys and exercises significant bureaucratic discretion. As a result, by the early 1990s, the program was generating approximately $500 million in savings per year,[48] and was doing so without adversely affecting beneficiary access or the quality of care provided.[49]

The only exception to California's hospital cost-containment regime occurred in the early 1990s, when two factors prompted a crisis. First, the number of uninsured state residents had risen to over 6 million. Second, the safety net hospitals (mainly county facilities and several large nonprofits) that treated the uninsured were in severe fiscal distress. After all, both Medi-Cal and Medicare, the two main sources of income for these hospitals, had instituted successful cost containment initiatives. Rather remarkably, however, there was suddenly a way for state officials to increase the reimbursement paid to the safety net hospitals without costing the state treasury a penny. Even California's cost-conscious bureaucrats could not resist this option.

The tale begins with the federal requirement that states provide additional reimbursement to hospitals that serve a disproportionate number of low-income patients. This federal program, enacted in 1981, was largely ignored until Congress pressured states to comply (in 1987), and states discovered that they could use provider taxes or voluntary donations to cover the state share of the increase. In 1991, California enacted a law requiring local hospital districts, the University of California, and county governments to pick up the entire state share of disproportionate share payments. As a result, if the state increased payment levels to disproportionate share hospitals by $100, the federal government paid $50 and local intergovernmental transfers covered the rest.

By 1993, California had the second largest disproportionate share program in the nation (behind only New York). Under the program, approximately 79 hospitals around the state received over $1.5 billion in disproportionate share payments.[50] The program was popular with the hospitals (which relied on the extra money for survival), with local governments (which received an infusion of federal dollars), and with state officials (who organized the fiscal maneuvering). The program allowed state officials to keep state Medi-Cal expenditures low while simultaneously responding to the needs of providers and local governments.

Viewed together, the selective contracting program and the disproportionate share program suggest an important lesson about California hospital politics: providers and local governments have only limited influence, and unions are not key players at all. More specifically, while state bureaucrats have the discretion to implement a comprehensive cost containment initiative, they are willing to maximize federal funds to support the providers and counties.

New York vs. California: Adding Up the Score

New York's Medicaid program spends more on inpatient hospital care than does California, even though it pays for fewer inpatient admissions. In fiscal year 1989, for example, New York's program spent $2.26 billion on 411,032 admissions while California spent $1.97 billion on 515,155 admissions.[51] More generally, New York in 1993 spent $7.3 billion on hospital care for its 2.7 million beneficiaries, while California spent $6.3 billion on 4.8 million recipients.[52] New York's program also pays a higher percentage of the actual cost of each admission than does California. In 1993, for example, New York's program paid on average 101 percent of actual cost while Medi-Cal paid 96 percent.[53]

There is an important caveat: the average cost per patient per day is much lower in New York than it is in California. This is true not just for Medicaid but across all payers. In 1992, for example, the cost per patient per day in New York (for all payers) was $819; in California it was $1,199.[54] Nonetheless, the average cost per admission is much higher in New York ($7,390 as opposed to $6,470 in California). This anomaly is due primarily to the tendency of New Yorkers to have longer lengths of stay (9.2 days in New York compared to 6.6 in California in 1992).[55]

Cost comparisons aside, it is clear that the policymaking environments in the two states differ substantially. In New York, inpatient reimbursement politics is set in a pluralistic environment: state officials, provider associations, union leaders, insurance executives, and consumer advocates all participate in and influence policy. In California, in contrast, inpatient reimbursement policy is established by an autonomous and centralized state agency, the California Medical Assistance Commission. Over half of California's hospitals no longer participate in Medi-Cal, and those that remain negotiate individual contracts in secret negotiations with state administrators. The contrast between the bureaucratic environments could not be sharper.

8

Moving Medicaid Clients into Managed Care

Managed Care Becomes Mainstream Care

While Congress debated whether and how to provide health insurance to the thirty-nine million uninsured, the health care system for the rest of the population underwent a remarkable transformation. No longer do most Americans have indemnity insurance policies, which cover medical care provided by any available doctor, and which pay the doctor a separate fee for every service performed.[1] Instead, Americans today increasingly belong to managed care organizations,[2] which not only limit consumer freedom of choice, but which also provide doctors with fiscal incentives to reduce the volume of health care.

The enthusiasm for managed care is especially apparent among those state officials who argue that encouraging (or requiring) Medicaid beneficiaries to enroll in managed care will simultaneously save money, improve access to care, and lead to better quality care. The argument is illustrated by the following hypothetical example. In 1994, state X spent $100 per month on an average Medicaid client. In 1995, the state pays participating health plans $95 to provide enrollees with a comprehensive set of medical benefits. State officials claim an immediate $5 in savings. Officials also expect that health plans will effectively manage beneficiary care, discouraging clients from expensive and often inappropriate emergency room care and encouraging clients to receive instead inexpensive and more appropriate primary care. The case management should reduce total health costs and thereby enable the state to pay even less money in 1996.

Managed care as cost containment only works, however, if the Medicaid program would have spent more on the beneficiary in the old fee-for-service world than it would by paying the health plan. Consider again the managed care initiative in hypothetical state X. Mary Smith, a Medicaid beneficiary, joins the GoodHealth HMO. GoodHealth is now responsible for the full cost of Mrs. Smith's care: if her care costs less than $95 per month, the plan makes money; if her care costs more than $95 per month, it loses. The state saves money, however, only if Medicaid would have spent more than $95 on Mrs. Smith were she not in managed care. Otherwise, the state would be paying GoodHealth more than it would have paid directly. So if Mrs. Smith is a low-cost client who would have cost the state only $80 per month in a fee-for-service world, then the state has actually lost $15. Unfortunately, this scenario is not unusual: health plans often market to low-cost clients and avoid the higher-risk, higher-cost beneficiary.

The problem of health plan selection bias (or adverse selection) is reduced (but not eliminated) if managed care becomes mandatory. The problem would be further reduced if states could more accurately predict the future cost of beneficiary care and adjust payment to plans accordingly, paying more for the high cost clients and less for the others. But managed care as cost containment is limited by other factors as well. First, well-run managed care plans spend time and money trying to alter beneficiaries' patterns of health care use. They hire new staff (from social workers to interpreters), provide additional services (from transportation services to special prenatal care programs), and then seek from the state additional reimbursement for these start-up costs. The payoff, a reduction in high-cost emergency room and inpatient utilization, often takes years to achieve.

Another factor limiting savings is that states incur start-up costs as they reorganize Medicaid bureaucracies and retrain workers: the administrative tasks involved in regulating managed care systems (from reviewing marketing materials to setting capitation rates) differ greatly from fee-for-service administration.

Third, the managed care initiatives to date have usually enrolled only mothers and their young children. This is the least costly Medicaid population, comprising approximately 70 percent of Medicaid beneficiaries but accounting for only 30 percent of Medicaid dollars spent. To be sure, some states are experimenting with managed care for the aged, the disabled, and other clients with special needs, such as the mentally ill, substance abusers, or the chronically ill, but these efforts are sporadic at best.

Finally, managed care cost containment doesn't necessarily lead to improved access and quality. One of the ways health plans can reduce costs is by limiting client access to care. In the hypothetical state X, for example, the GoodHealth HMO receives $95 for Mrs. Smith's care regardless of how much care is actually provided. The fiscal incentive, as such, is to provide as little care as possible.

Despite the questions about Medicaid managed care, nearly every state is now encouraging its beneficiaries to enroll in managed care.[3] As a result, the number of Medicaid clients in managed care has grown from 750,000 in 1983 (3 percent of all enrollees) to 7.8 million in 1994 (23 percent of all enrollees).[4] Two of the largest managed care initiatives are in New York and California, and in this chapter I compare and contrast these programs. I begin with a historical overview of Medicaid managed care in the two states, focusing first on the period before 1991 (the era before the current managed care initiatives) and then on the initiatives now underway. I then contrast the extent to which the states have implemented policies to protect the medical safety net.[5] I conclude that California's initiative is less decentralized and pluralistic than New York's, and that California has used its discretion to adopt a strategy designed in large part to protect safety-net hospitals.

California in the 1970s: Managed Care Scandals and a Crumbling Safety Net

Beginning in the late 1960s, California officials initiated a large-scale effort to enroll Medi-Cal clients into managed care organizations. The effort, the first of its sort in the nation, was intended to reduce rising Medi-Cal costs: each participating HMO received, for every client it enrolled, a fee set at 80 percent of the cost of an average Medi-Cal client. In exchange, the HMOs both supplied clients with all required care and bore the fiscal risk for cost overruns.

California was (and is) a good state in which to test the viability of Medicaid managed care. Californians have long enrolled in managed care organizations, such as the Kaiser-Permanente health clinics, in numbers far greater than their counterparts in other states.[6] Given the state's large managed care industry, state officials argued both that mainstream care in California is managed care and that the state had the managed care infrastructure to accommodate the expansionary effort.

There was a problem, however: the managed care capitation rates were extraordinarily low, arguably too low to attract health plan participation. The low rates were due, in part, to the state's successful effort to contain Medi-Cal fee-for-service reimbursement levels: the low fee-for-service reimbursement meant low per beneficiary expenditures, which meant low managed care rates. The low rates were also due to bureaucratic design: indeed, while Governor Ronald Reagan suggested that Medi-Cal cost savings would come from the competition between private sector health plans, the real savings, if any, would come from the tightly regulated reimbursement formulas.

To counter the unattractively low rates, state officials offered the managed care community an informal deal: although rates would be low, there also would be minimal state oversight of health plan activity (this was the model used to keep nursing home reimbursement low). It soon became clear, however, that the mainstream managed care organizations were not interested in enrolling large numbers of Medi-Cal clients. One reason was the low rates: HMOs like Kaiser, which operated high-quality facilities, were pessimistic about their ability to operate a profitable Medi-Cal operation. Many mainstream plans were also concerned that enrolling Medi-Cal clients could encourage commercially insured clients to disenroll, particularly if the organization enrolled more than a token number of Medi-Cal clients.

With the mainstream managed care organizations reluctant to participate, businessmen and entrepreneurs created virtually overnight dozens of new managed care entities, which competed among themselves for the Medi-Cal clientele. The operators of many of these new entities had little or no experience as medical providers, but they were attracted by the promise of guaranteed income and the lack of state regulatory oversight. They began to market their wares door-to-door in low-income communities. Soon tens of thousands of Medi-Cal clients were signing up.

The emphasis on managed care posed a serious threat to the county hospital system, which at that time provided medical services to a majority of Medi-Cal clients. To be sure, the county system was already under siege. In 1971, for example, the state (in yet another cost-containment effort) dramatically increased the county share of Medi-Cal costs while simultaneously eliminating a program that helped counties pay for the cost of caring for the uninsured. These changes imposed significant fiscal stress on the counties and led several to either close or scale back their county hospitals. At the same time, however, the managed care initiative was diverting Medi-Cal clients away from county facilities, leaving these facilities to care for an increasingly uninsured population. And when Medi-Cal clients sought care from county hospital emergency rooms, rather than from their new managed care "gatekeeper" (as many clients did), the managed care organization (and Medi-Cal itself) would generally reject claims for reimbursement, undermining further the already precarious state of these facilities.

With the county safety net crumbling, more and more Medi-Cal clients joined the new managed care organizations. Soon, however, many of the new organizations were embroiled in controversy and scandal. There were at least four problems. First, many of the organizations relied on unlawful marketing techniques. Some door-to-door marketers, for example, told clients that enrollment was mandatory (it wasn't). Others promised benefits and perks well beyond the Medicaid package. Second, client access to care was often inadequate, particularly after normal working hours. Moreover, even when clients did get an appointment, they often waited hours for poor quality care. (It was hardly surprising that many clients soon returned to the county hospital emergency room.) Third, client efforts to disenroll were often ignored, or at the least excessively delayed. Fourth, and finally, many of the new organizations were inadequately capitalized (some went bankrupt rather quickly), while others were rife with fraud and profiteering.

In the early 1970s, in response to the crisis, California's legislature enacted a series of incremental efforts to regulate the newly emerging managed care organizations.[7] Around that same time, federal investigators reported the problems with California's managed care initiative and suggested that Congress should regulate Medicaid managed care programs.[8] Shortly thereafter, Congress enacted the Health Maintenance Organization Amendments of 1976, which imposed significant federal restrictions on state managed care initiatives. The law required, for example, that only federally qualified HMOs could receive full-risk Medicaid contracts. The law required also that no more than 50 percent of any HMO's clientele be Medicaid or Medicare recipients (thus virtually eliminating the "Medicaid-only" HMO).[9] Since few of the new Medicaid HMOs were federally qualified, and since most had more than 50 percent Medicaid enrollees, the new federal legislation (together with the tightened state regulation) ended California's early experiment with Medicaid managed care. By the late 1970s, for example, the number of managed care organizations with Medi-Cal contracts had declined, from sixty-five to twenty-one.

As the managed care initiative ended, Medi-Cal clients again sought care from the county hospital safety net. But the counties were ill-equipped to respond to the rise in utilization. Rising health care costs had prompted counties to raise property taxes, and rising property taxes had encouraged the tax revolt of 1978 (otherwise known as Proposition 13), which both rolled back property tax levels and sharply limited future increases.

The state, which at that time had the luxury of a $3.7 billion budget surplus, responded to the counties fiscal crisis by assuming the counties' share of Medi-Cal expenditures and by enacting the County Health Services Fund (which provided state funds for county health costs). The pendulum had shifted: the managed care initiative was over (though a few managed care contracts remained in place), and the emphasis instead was on restoring the fiscal health of the county health system.

California in the 1980s: Incremental Growth in Medicaid Managed Care

When Ronald Reagan was elected president in 1980, he decided that the Medicaid program should delegate more authority to the states and that states should be encouraged to experiment with managed care initiatives. As a result, federal legislation in 1981 increased significantly state discretion over Medicaid policy and loosened significantly federal restrictions on Medicaid managed care programs. For example, nonfederally qualified HMOs could now receive full-risk Medicaid contracts, the rule that required HMOs to have no more than 50 percent Medicaid and Medicare clients was amended upward to 75 percent, and states were authorized to offer six months of guaranteed eligibility to those Medicaid clients who enrolled in managed care.

The changed federal environment was particularly appreciated in California, which was then suffering from a severe recession, the cost of the county bailout, and a decline in federal aid. The state's budget surplus was gone, replaced by a budget deficit, and the state in 1982 enacted a major Medi-Cal reform package. The 1982 reforms are best known for requiring hospitals to bid for Medi-Cal contracts (the so-called selective contracting system).[10] But the legislation also followed the federal lead and authorized some incremental expansions in Medi-Cal's now small managed care program. The new efforts fell into two categories. First, there were efforts to encourage clients to enroll voluntarily in the new Primary Care Case Management Program (PCCM). This program provided doctors with a fixed fee both for providing primary care services to enrollees and for supervising client efforts to receive specialty care. The expectation was that, over time, participating providers would become full-risk prepaid plans.

Second, the 1982 legislation authorized three counties to require local Medi-Cal clients to enroll in managed care. Two of these counties, Santa Barbara and Monterey, received permission to operate County Organized Health Systems (COHSs). The COHSs in these counties would receive from the state a fixed fee for every local Medi-Cal resident. The COHS would then contract with local providers to care for the Medi-Cal population. Medi-Cal clients were required to belong to the COHS, and the COHS served only the Medi-Cal population.[11] The third county aided by the 1982 legislation, San Diego, received permission to require its Medi-Cal clients to pick from a menu of private managed care plans.

Despite the renewed interest in Medicaid managed care, the new initiatives proceeded slowly. The Monterey COHS was abandoned shortly after it started, a victim of poor planning and inadequate funding. San Diego's effort to require Medi-Cal clients to choose from a menu of managed care plans was undermined by the California Medical Association, which protested that the plan would disrupt the medical care received by thousands of senior citizens. And only one PCCM provider ever became a full-risk provider, despite the state's hope that all of the nearly two dozen such providers would do so.

There were also complaints, by both consumer advocates and

some state officials, about the quality of care provided by the PCCMs. First, there were numerous anecdotal reports of PCCMs providing poor access to care (long waits for appointments, no evening appointments, and so on). Second, there were suggestions that some PCCMs discouraged necessary inpatient care (since they got a fiscal bonus for reducing such care). And third, the state had very little regulatory control over PCCM behavior, since the Knox-Keene legislation of 1975 (which governed HMOs) did not cover PCCMs.

Perhaps the only success stories of the 1980s initiatives were the COHSs in Santa Barbara and San Mateo (the San Mateo COHS was authorized in 1983 and began operations in 1987). By all accounts, the two programs have cut costs, both by cutting client inpatient utilization and by persuading primary care providers to reduce specialist referrals. Moreover, clients and providers alike generally consider the programs to be unusually consumer friendly.

Despite the success of the COHS model, however, the number of Medi-Cal clients enrolled in managed care increased only incrementally during the 1980s (reaching approximately 355,000 by 1990).[12] As in the 1970s, a key problem was the state's success in keeping regular Medicaid rates (based on a fee-for-service methodology) quite low. Since managed care rates are required by law to be less than the fee-for-service rates, finding (reputable) plans willing to accept the necessarily low capitation rate was particularly difficult.

At the same time, the state's governor during much of the 1980s, George Dukemedjian, had little interest in health care policy. Dukemedjian's priorities were cutting taxes, building prisons, and shrinking social welfare programs. He had little interest in challenging the California Medical Association, for example, when it opposed the San Diego managed care initiative. Under his leadership, state health officials avoided major new initiatives, and the Medi-Cal delivery system remained predominantly fee-for-service.

California in the 1990s: A Renewed Emphasis on Managed Care

By the early 1990s, rising Medicaid costs persuaded California officials of the desirability of a renewed emphasis on managed care. The newly elected governor, Pete Wilson, supported the effort, and in 1991 the state legislature, in the waning moments of the legislative session, enacted a new Medi-Cal managed care initiative. That the legislation was pushed through by the administration with little debate or discussion caused concern among the traditional opponents of managed care (the counties, the doctors, and the consumer advocates), but the initiative was sufficiently incremental that the opposition was relatively muted. For example, the legislation authorized three new COHSs, hardly a surprise since Congress the previous year had itself authorized the limited COHS expansion. The legislation also allowed a revised version of the San Diego managed care experiment (now called geographic managed care) in two counties. Finally, and most controversially, it required that Medi-Cal clients who do not affirmatively choose a fee-for-service physician be enrolled into managed care by default.

The task of implementing the new legislation was assigned primarily to the California Department of Health Services (DHS), the state agency generally in charge of the Medi-Cal program. The California Medical Assistance Commission (CMAC), created in 1982 to administer the hospital selective contracting program, was to work with DHS in implementing both the new COHS efforts and the new geographic managed care program.

In early 1992, DHS established a goal of expanding the number of Medi-Cal clients in managed care from 530,000 (or about 11 percent of the total Medi-Cal enrollment) to 1.25 million (27 percent of the total) by early 1997. DHS then decided that to meet this goal it would (1) ensure that the presentation to clients at the time of enrollment emphasized managed care; (2) implement the default enrollment by early 1994; (3) authorize managed care plans to provide nonmonetary incentives to prospective enrollees; (4) expand the PCCM program; (5) encourage HMOs to accept Medi-Cal clients; (6) provide case management for high-cost clients; and (7) work with CMAC in developing the new COHS and geographic managed care programs.

Almost immediately, the implementation effort ran into problems. There was significant interest group opposition to the initiative, and DHS at that time (and in this policy arena) lacked the bureaucratic autonomy to overcome the opposition. Legal services lawyers, for example, challenged the legality of the new default program.[13] HMOs were still reluctant to accept Medi-Cal clients. Most importantly, counties (particularly the larger ones) were not only reluctant to participate in either the COHS or geographic managed care experiments, they were opposed to the entire initiative.

County opposition to managed care had grown increasingly sharp, partly as the result of state legislation enacted in 1991, under which state aid for county health programs was discontinued, county responsibility for indigent health care was expanded, and counties were given additional tax revenue (primarily from the state sales tax) to make up for the lost revenue. Even in the best of economic times the counties would have lost money under the new division of responsibility, but with the severe recession resulting both in reduced sales tax revenue and increased demands on the county safety net, many counties soon faced a severe fiscal crisis.

Fortunately for the counties, however, the federal program that required states to provide additional reimbursement to those hospitals that treat a disproportionate share of low-income persons was at the same time providing county hospitals with hundreds of millions of dollars in supplemental Medi-Cal payments.[14] The county hospitals used the increased reimbursement to recoup lost state funds and to care for the uninsured more generally. But if the Medi-Cal population moved primarily into private HMOs, the county hospitals would lose not only much of their insured clientele, but also their disproportionate-share funding. The counties would be left with a predominately uninsured patient base and with inadequate funding to subsidize their care.

Given the county opposition, the state was unable to persuade any counties to volunteer for the geographic managed care initiative. State officials eventually required Sacramento County to participate in the demonstration. State officials also had a difficult time finding volunteers for the COHSs program. Finally, three counties without county hospitals (Orange, Santa Cruz, and Solano) agreed to participate.

A few months later, in July 1992, the surprisingly pluralistic politics of Medi-Cal managed care changed again when a large for-profit HMO, the Foundation Health Plan, claimed that it could cover the entire Medi-Cal population and save the state hundreds of millions of dollars while doing so.

Foundation's bid for an exclusive Medi-Cal contract received support from influential legislators (most prominently Willie Brown) and from state budget officials. But the bid was opposed by nearly every interested interest group,[15] and by the state's Medicaid agency (DHS) as well. Hospitals (both public and private) worried about losing patients and disproportionate share funding. HMOs worried that a competitor would accumulate several million new clients (even though they had little interest in such clients themselves). Doctors worried about a large-scale shift to managed care. Community clinics and other small safety net providers worried about losing their primary source of income. Consumer advocates worried that Foundation would provide Medi-Cal clients with poor quality health care. The California Medical Assistance Commission worried that if Foundation succeeded, the COHS model, which it supported (and administered), would soon decline. And state Medi-Cal officials (in the DHS) worried about losing control of the program itself.

As part of its effort to defeat the Foundation bid, DHS officials began a campaign to demonstrate that it too could rapidly increase the state's managed care capacity. During the summer of 1992, for example, DHS proposed legislation that would require that 5 percent of every HMO's client population be Medi-Cal clients. While the California Association of HMOs strongly opposed the 5 percent mandate, its members agreed (in the so-called CAHMO Agreement) to accept an additional hundred thousand Medi-Cal clients.[16] DHS also persuaded the California Association of Public Hospitals to not only promise to create lots of new publicly operated managed care organizations, but also to suggest that the new organizations could enroll over one million Medi-Cal clients. And DHS increased its effort to persuade small groups of physicians either to join the Primary Care Case Management Program or to provide other forms of Medi-Cal case management.

In the end, the coalition opposed to the Foundation bid was strong enough to defeat it. But in September 1992 the legislature enacted a bill that both required DHS to speed up the transition to managed care and provided DHS with significant discretion in meeting that goal. For example, the legislation authorized DHS to enact "emergency" managed care regulations without going through normal notice and comment procedures. Perhaps ironically, the same forces that coalesced to defeat the Foundation bid also led (albeit unintentionally) to a dramatic increase in DHS authority.

To be sure, interest group influence hardly disappeared simply because DHS had increased bureaucratic discretion. Medi-Cal director Molly Coye even promised that DHS would work closely with all interested parties in directing the movement toward managed care. Even as Dr. Coye spoke, however, her staff was developing an aggressive and ambitious expansion program, one which focused both on expanding the Primary Care Case Management Program and on encouraging more private sector HMOs to accept Medi-Cal clients. DHS staff placed less of an emphasis on expanding public sector managed care programs, including both the public hospitals' initiative and the COHS approach.

The tension between the pluralistic politics that Dr. Coye acknowledged and the bureaucratic control her colleagues pursued reached a fever pitch in October 1992, when Santa Clara officials learned, after the fact, that DHS staff had signed a contract with PruCare, a large Primary Care Case Management program, to provide care to Medi-Cal clients in Santa Clara County. The PruCare contract mobilized the counties and the consumer advocates: not only would the contract undercut the county hospital and other safety net providers, but PruCare itself was an organization often accused of providing poor quality care and engaging in marketing abuses. Indeed, and rather ironically, DHS released a report critical of PruCare's activities in southern California just as the agency was signing the contract with PruCare in Santa Clara.

In response to the political uproar generated by the PruCare contract, Dr. Coye, in November 1992, declared a moratorium on new managed care contracts. She also asked several of her staff to develop and defend a more formal managed care policy (and to do so within a couple of months). If DHS was to effectively wrest control of the managed care policy arena, it needed a more thoughtful organizational position and a more consistent bureaucratic message.

During the managed care moratorium, several key interest groups sought to influence the DHS position. The physician community favored an expanded COHS program, as did the California Medical Assistance Commission (which hoped to supervise any new COHSs), several large counties (which hoped to make the best of a bad situation), and most consumer advocates. At the same time, many in the HMO industry, along with many on the right of the political spectrum, argued that a COHS was a single-payer system in disguise, vesting far too much authority in governmental bureaucracy. The HMOs and the conservatives favored an expansion of the geographic managed care program, under which several health plans could compete for Medi-Cal business.

DHS generally ignored the interest groups. Agency officials instead released a draft managed care initiative on January 13, 1994 that proposed an entirely new managed care structure: "interested parties" in eleven of the state's largest counties would develop "health care consortia," which would offer Medi-Cal clients a choice of managed care plans. By July 1994, 2.4 million Medi-Cal clients would be enrolled in managed care, an increase from 606,000.

Given the large number of groups interested in the managed care initiative, DHS officials did, however, take their proposal on the road, holding hearings and soliciting written comments. Group after group criticized the plan. The counties argued that the consortia model was a COHS without the counties in charge (indeed, it was impossible to tell who would be in charge of forming and administering the consortia), and that the proposal inadequately protected disproportionate share funds received by county hospitals. HMOs and other providers objected to a requirement that organizations in the consortia had to drop any rate-related lawsuit brought against the state. Advocates argued that the proposal relied too heavily on private sector HMOs and PCCMs. The California Medical Assistance Commission complained that it had been given too small of an administrative role. And nearly every group suggested that the plan contained unrealistic time frames (for example, "interested parties" had less than four months to form a consortium).

Given the negative response, DHS retreated and reevaluated its plan. At the same time, however, DHS itself was questioning the wisdom of delegating significant authority to a sole source (whether called a consortium, a COHS, or something else). DHS's concern was prompted by an ongoing rate dispute with the San Mateo COHS. The dispute began in early 1992 when a state audit claimed that San Mateo's reserves were too high, and that its reimbursement rate was too high as well.[17] State officials then demanded a significant rate reduction.[18] In response, Mike Murray, the San Mateo CEO, threatened to shut down the entire San Mateo operation. Murray's threat enabled San Mateo to negotiate a more favorable deal. It also persuaded many DHS officials that an expanded managed care initiative should avoid sole source contracts.

In an effort to decide on a new strategy, DHS assigned six staffers to spend six weeks in a "hideaway location" and instructed them not to emerge until a final plan was in place.[19] The goal (again) was to limit interest group influence. As before, the insulation strategy succeeded, and the staffers developed a completely new idea, the so-called two-plan model. This innovative managed care initiative has five key features. First, twelve of the state's largest counties will develop a "local initiative," or a government run HMO.[20] But to ensure competition (and to avoid another San Mateo), there will also be in each county a "mainstream" or private sector plan. Second, the private sector plan can be either a single HMO (like the Foundation Health Plan) or a joint venture with several HMOs. Third, the government-run plan will be guaranteed a minimum number of Medi-Cal clients (so as to protect county hospital disproportionate care funding). Fourth, when the new system is in place (in late 1996), PCCMs will no longer be licensed, and HMO enrollees must join one of the two plans. Fifth, and finally, DHS (and not CMAC) will administer the new system.

DHS officials insist that the new approach will reduce the state's administrative burden, eliminate excessive competition, and protect safety-net providers (primarily by preserving disproportionate-share funding). The officials are, as of this writing, pushing ahead with their implementation time frame. In October 1995, DHS awarded mainstream plan contracts in all but one of the twelve counties. In Los Angeles, for example, Foundation Health Plan received the contract, defeating three other bidders. The state expects most mainstream plans to begin operations by late 1996. At the same time, DHS is working with counties as they plan and develop local initiatives.

The interest-group opposition to the initiative remains strong. The most vocal opponents are the HMOs (especially those that bid and lost). The HMOs object to the decision to permit only one private-sector plan in each county and to the requirement that the local initiative be guaranteed a minimum number of clients. The HMOs also complain about the state's efforts to keep capitation rates low. Unlike New York, where there is near parity in the public and private rates, current Medi-Cal capitation rates are about 33 percent less than the average commercial rates,[21] there is a three-year freeze on such rates, and the rates proposed for two-plan model participants are lower still. The low rates raise again the memories of the 1970s, when bargain basement managed care rates encouraged bargain basement managed care plans. Even federal officials worry that the rates may be too low.[22]

At the same time, the counties, though more supportive of the two-plan model, argue that private-sector plans are using the transition period to enroll scores of low-risk beneficiaries, leaving the high-risk (and more expensive) clients for the evolving public plans. Physicians worry that existing physician-patient relationships will be disrupted and that client care will suffer. Small safety net clinics fear that they might not survive the transition to managed care, and consumer advocates complain about the speed with which the state is proceeding. As of October 1994, for example, there were only 927,000 Medi-Cal beneficiaries enrolled in managed care; the state plans to triple that number by late 1996.

Along with the interest-group opposition, there are intergovernmental obstacles as well. Specifically, mandatory enrollment under the two-plan model cannot begin until and unless authorized by the federal Health Care Financing Administration (HCFA), and HCFA approval is still in doubt. One problem is a 1994 HCFA report suggesting that the state is moving too fast and that it lacks the resources (from staff to data systems) to supervise the transition adequately.[23] Another red flag was raised by a 1995 General Accounting Office report that criticized both the two-plan model itself (for restricting competition) and the state's managed care oversight capacity.[24] Given this criticism, the waiver approval process may not be resolved for several more months.

Finally, there is also controversy over the efforts of DHS to freeze out the California Medical Assistance Commission, especially since the commission is well-versed in administering managed care plans. Clearly, maintaining and expanding its bureaucratic autonomy is a high priority for DHS. Given this mission, the decision by DHS to push ahead with the two-plan model, despite interest-group and intergovernmental opposition, is hardly surprising. Moreover, the state-dominated initiative emerging today contrasts sharply with the decentralized and fragmented initiative now underway in New York.

New York in the 1970s: Managed Care as Afterthought

During the 1970s and early 1980s, only twenty thousand of New York's two million Medicaid beneficiaries were enrolled in managed care, and nearly all of them were in a single plan, the Health Insurance Plan of New York (HIP). One reason for this was the low managed care penetration rate in the state generally. In 1984, fewer than one million New Yorkers were enrolled in managed care. State policy before 1985 even prohibited investor-owned HMOs from operating in New York.[25]

A second reason for the paltry enrollment in Medicaid managed care was the influential interest-group opposition. New York City's public hospitals and academic medical centers relied heavily on Medicaid funds received for emergency room care; an emphasis on managed care would substantially reduce those funds. Organized labor worried that if managed care hurt the hospital sector, non-professional health care workers would be the first to lose their jobs. Consumer advocates argued that managed care would reduce access to care, citing the California scandals as evidence.

Third, the state's Medicaid reimbursement patterns, well-established by the early 1970s, were decidedly hostile to a managed care initiative. More than any other state, New York's program has long favored institution-based specialty care and disfavored the community-based primary care needed for a managed care network.

New York ranks fiftieth among the states in the ratio of Medicaid physician fees to both Medicare-allowed charges and private fees,[26] providing the absurdly low sum of $11 for a routine office visit.[27] At the same time, however, New York pays skilled nursing facilities more than twice the national average,[28] pays more than $6,000 per Medicaid client for inpatient hospital care (the third highest among the states),[29] and manages itself to spend nearly 16 percent of the nation's entire Medicaid budget. Managed care cannot thrive if revenues are directed away from primary care gatekeepers and toward specialists and institutions.

The rocky politics of Medicaid managed care during this era is illustrated by the disappointing efforts to initiate mandatory managed care programs in two very different communities: northern Manhattan and Rochester.

The New York City story began in 1980, when Mayor Ed Koch proposed closing two large public hospitals (Sydenham and Metropolitan). The proposal was fiercely opposed by leaders in the African-American community, labor unions, physicians, and the Catholic Church. As a compromise, Koch suggested that Sydenham be replaced by a collection of ambulatory clinics and that Metropolitan be replaced by a city-run HMO, called CitiCaid, which would be mandatory for local Medicaid beneficiaries and available to the local uninsured. Koch's opponents were equally opposed to a mandatory managed care program, however, arguing that it discriminated against poor (and mainly minority) beneficiaries. Koch backtracked again, proposing that CitiCaid be a purely voluntary program. Only then did the opposition lessen, and in September 1985 the program accepted its first enrollees.

The enactment of CitiCaid did not, however, persuade city officials of the merits of managed care. To the contrary, city officials, worried about the fiscal health of the public hospital system, generally opposed managed care. Indeed, even though CitiCaid seemed to work well, providing a delivery system model now replicated by a couple of states, it remained a small and largely ignored program.

The Rochester story began in 1982 when federal officials decided that Monroe County (comprised primarily of Rochester) could participate in a federal demonstration program designed to test the viability of mandatory Medicaid managed care. Three years later, in late 1985, more than twenty thousand clients were participating. By late 1986 the figure was well over forty thousand.

Just a year later, however, in late 1987, the program (called Medi-Cap) was dismantled.[30]

The proximate cause of Medi-Cap's demise was the state's decision, in mid-1986, to reduce the program's capitation rate by 12 percent, which in turn led several of the participating providers to drop out.[31] But the real problem was that too much money was spent on program administration, while too little was spent educating providers (few of whom were HMOs) on the mechanics of managing care.

The Medi-Cap Corporation, for example, that administered the program (under regulations set by various state and federal agencies) received from Medicaid a capitation rate of approximately 95 percent of the fee-for-service expenditures of an average Medicaid client. The Corporation then paid the Rochester Health Network (RHN), a large local HMO, approximately 94 percent of the amount it received. RHN in turn paid the actual providers (mainly nine community health centers) 90 to 92 percent of the money it received. The end result: the community health centers bore the full risk for their clients' care for just over 80 percent of the fee-for-service rate. Moreover, the health centers themselves generally offered only primary care: when clients needed to see specialists or enter the hospital, the centers generally paid the market rate.[32]

Most of the participating health centers were neither sophisticated financially nor experienced at managing care. They were ill-equipped to handle the dramatic client expansion, particularly when so much of the capitation rate was absorbed by larger administrative entities. But unlike many California HMOs that in the 1970s provided poor care for poor rates, Rochester's health centers tried to provide good care for poor rates. It didn't work.

New York in the 1980s: Managed Care Moves onto the Agenda

Despite the demise of the mandatory managed care experiments, many state officials continued to support managed care as a strategy to combat Medicaid's rising hospital bill. Given the strong anti–managed care coalition, however, a successful managed care initiative needed to be incremental, voluntary, and nonthreatening to safety net hospitals. In this context, the state legislature in 1984 provided start-up funds for safety net providers to form prepaid health services plans (PHSPs), a new type of HMO that could enroll Medicaid and other publicly funded beneficiaries but could not compete in the commercial market. The policy assumption was that safety-net hospitals would form PHSPs, which would compete for Medicaid clients, and that revenue lost by the emergency room would be recovered by the health plans. The legislation authorized seven PHSPs. Nearly thirty organizations applied for the state start-up funds; eight were funded, and five programs were eventually implemented.

To be sure, the legislation also authorized counties to establish Physician Case Management Programs, under which individual physicians would receive enhanced fees in exchange for serving as managed care gatekeepers. This program resembled California's Primary Care Case Management Program. But the state neither provided start-up funds for this initiative, nor encouraged counties to participate. Not surprisingly, only one county (Erie) signed up.

The PHSP program did have some success stories. For example, the director of ambulatory care at Montefiore Hospital converted three hospital clinics into a thriving PHSP called the Bronx Health Plan, which by late 1993 served approximately twenty-five thousand members, 90 percent of whom are Medicaid clients.[33] Other PHSPs have also done well financially, despite receiving, for every beneficiary enrolled, less than 90 percent of the cost of an average Medicaid client. One reason for the success is that New York's fee-for-service costs are quite high, so a capitation rate based on those rates is also high. For example, New York's HMOs receive from Medicaid $140 to $160 per month for an average child, a rate that is on par with that paid by most commercial payers. A California HMO, in contrast, receives from Medi-Cal $80 to $100 per month for a similarly situated child, a rate much less than regular commercial rates.[34]

Despite the success of the PHSPs, the program itself never generated the hoped-for hospital participation. Indeed, most of the PHSPs emerged from small community health centers and not from large acute care hospitals, and most did not develop until the early 1990s. The small incentive of state start-up funds was insufficient to lure most hospitals into the uncharted waters of Medicaid managed care.

But although the hospital industry hoped to maintain the status quo, the HMO industry anticipated major marketplace changes. Several of the nation's large for-profit HMOs accelerated their efforts to enter the New York State market. The legal basis for their exclusion was tenuous: state officials interpreted a law that excluded investor-owned hospitals to exclude also investor-owned HMOs, even though HMOs were governed by an entirely different set of state laws. With the HMOs threatening litigation, and state officials themselves questioning the exclusion, the Health Department in 1985 changed its policy and permitted investor-owned HMOs to enter the state. Given the growing interest in Medicaid managed care, however, the department added a requirement that the newly licensed HMOs must "demonstrate a willingness" to enroll Medicaid clients. But not surprisingly, few commercial HMOs were interested in the Medicaid population (their goal instead was to tap into the state's lucrative and growing private market), and the state did little to enforce its new (and vague) regulation.

With the 1984 Medicaid managed care initiative lagging, and with the newly licensed commercial HMOs generally avoiding Medicaid clients, New York's policy environment was drifting away from its flirtation with Medicaid managed care. The drift ended, however, when the New York City Task Force on Medicaid recommended that New York City itself should adopt a mandatory managed care demonstration project. The proposal, like the earlier CitiCaid initiative, was sharply attacked by hospitals, unions, and advocates. Once again, city officials proposed a compromise: a pilot project in a small section of southwest Brooklyn. This time, however, the state legislature, unhappy with the progress of the 1984 initiative, was willing to authorize the demonstration, especially since the city seemed anxious and committed.

The 1988 legislation also provided start-up funds for county-based Physician Case Management Programs, and it established a program (called Utilization Thresholds) under which clients who "overused" the medical system would be assigned a case manager. Nonetheless, the managed care evolution remained incremental: the southwest Brooklyn project was limited to twenty-five thousand enrollees; the Physician Case Management Program was still small; and there was no real effort to encourage HMOs to accept Medicaid clients. By the end of the 1980s, there were still less than fifty-thousand Medicaid clients enrolled in managed care.

New York in the 1990s: Managed Care Takes Center Stage

In June 1991, the state legislature enacted a sweeping managed care initiative, declaring that 50 percent of the state's 2.5 million Medicaid clients would be enrolled in managed care before the end of the decade. With only seventy-five thousand clients then in managed care, the initiative promised to revolutionize the state's Medicaid program. Surprisingly, however, the bill generated relatively little opposition: none of the consumer advocates, public hospital officials, or labor leaders lobbied hard against the proposal. Their acquiescence, though unexpected, was attributable to four factors.

First, the movement toward managed care was sweeping Medicaid programs around the country. With program costs rising nearly 30 percent a year, and with clients still receiving most of their care in hospital emergency rooms, the idea of managed care seemed irresistible. Clients would receive better and less expensive care. Who could say no, particularly since the alternatives (cutting eligibility, benefits, or provider reimbursement) seemed so unattractive.

Second, the legislation delegated to the counties the task of developing a plan to enroll local Medicaid clients into managed care programs. The delegation of authority persuaded county leaders (and public hospital officials) that local interests would not be ignored. A county could, for example, encourage (or require) a local public hospital to participate. It could encourage HMOs to be active participants. Or it could build on local provider networks of all sorts to develop the delivery system.

The decision to delegate also enabled state legislators to sidestep some particularly difficult policy quandaries. The safety net hospitals, for example, urged that HMOs be required to reimburse hospitals when an HMO client receives nonurgent care in an emergency room. After all, not only are emergency rooms required by law to treat all who seek care, but the Medicaid reimbursement rate for an emergency room visit ($95) is much less than the cost of treating a true emergency. But the HMO lobby insisted that managed care works only if clients stop using emergency rooms inappropriately, and that paying for nonurgent care reinforces all the wrong incentives. The legislature, however, instead of resolving the emergency room reimbursement debate, delegated it to the counties.

Third, the legislation phased in managed care over several years. The transition had two parts. Counties would have three years to develop their own managed care plans: nineteen of the state's fifty-seven counties would develop a plan in year one, nineteen in year two, and the last nineteen in year three. This timing enabled those counties most ready for managed care to move quickly, but gave more time to others. Moreover, each plan had to meet phased-in targets: 10 percent of enrollees should be in managed care after one year, 25 percent after three, and 50 percent after five. This timing enabled counties to plan long-term for how best to accomplish the transition.

Fourth, and most important, the transition to managed care would be voluntary, at least unless a particular county decided otherwise (and received federal permission to do so). The southwest Brooklyn demonstration project would remain the state's only mandatory managed care initiative. Medicaid clients elsewhere would be encouraged, but not required, to enroll in managed care. To be sure, most analysts (including those in the state's Department of Social Services) doubted that a purely voluntary program would reach the 50 percent target. But the claim that a managed care initiative would inevitably restrict client freedom of choice was, for the time being anyway, removed from the debate.

The more immediate problem was to develop a managed care infrastructure to accommodate the new enrollees. The counties could require public hospitals to develop a managed care capacity, but they lacked similar leverage over the HMO community. While HMOs were required by law to show "a willingness" to accept Medicaid clients, the provision was too vague to be effective.

Perhaps surprisingly, however, HMOs were soon competing fiercely for the Medicaid business. Some observers attributed the change to a state law, enacted in early 1992, that imposed a 9 percent surcharge on the hospital bills of those HMOs that have too few Medicaid clients.[35] Without doubt, the surcharge was a factor: several HMOs accepted their first Medicaid clients only because they had to. But the HMOs continued to enroll large numbers of Medicaid clients even after a federal court held that the surcharge violated the federal Employee Retirement Income and Security Act (ERISA).[36]

The better explanation is that HMOs now understand the economic rationale for enrolling Medicaid clients. Medicaid in New York is a generous payer and enrolling Medicaid clients generates profits. The high rates have two explanations. First, managed care rates are based on Medicaid fee-for-service costs, and New York's fee-for-service costs are more than twice the national average. Second, managed care rates are developed through direct negotiations between state officials and health plan officials. Such plan-specific rates are unusual; most states set a single rate for all plans (with adjustments for the age, gender, and residence of the beneficiary) or determine rates according to a competitive bidding process. New York officials, however, negotiate rates with plan representatives once a year.

In this changing Medicaid marketplace, the safety net hospitals (particularly New York City's public hospitals) are forced to compete as well. One option is to persuade HMOs to refer patients to their facilities. But most HMOs prefer to contract with low-cost voluntary hospitals. The public hospitals must instead become managed care entities and compete directly for Medicaid enrollees. New York City's Health and Hospitals Corporation (HHC), for example, which administers the city's eleven acute care hospitals, determined that its economic viability depended on how successfully it expanded its managed care capacity. Other safety-net hospitals reached a similar conclusion.

Given the sudden competition for Medicaid business, the numbers of clients enrolled in managed care expanded significantly, from 62,000 in early 1991 to more than 600,000 in early 1995 (or 24 percent of the eligible population). All fifty-seven of the state's counties have exceeded their enrollment targets. The managed care initiative seems to be working so well that newly elected Republican Governor George Pataki has requested permission from the federal government to require (almost) all beneficiaries to enroll in managed care within the next two years.

The rapid growth of Medicaid managed care raises important political questions. Is managed care politics in New York still pluralistic, or are state officials able now to exercise greater policymaking discretion? Why are the traditional opponents of managed care (the hospitals, unions, and advocates) unable or unwilling to slow the growth? How influential has the HMO industry become?

It may take several years before answers to these questions are clear. Governor Pataki, for example, is trying hard to increase the state's role: not only has he proposed mandatory managed care for most Medicaid beneficiaries, he also hopes to have HMOs bid for managed care contracts, and to end the system of separately negotiated capitation rates. For now, however, pluralism and decentralization remain the trademarks of New York's Medicaid managed care initiative. Managed care enrollment is still voluntary (in almost all of the state). Managed care policy is set largely by the fifty-seven counties. Rates are still set on a case-by-case basis, after bargaining and negotiation. The rates themselves are unusually high. Many managed care plans compete, including several that serve only Medicaid clients. The marketing and enrollment process has largely been unregulated. Neither the state nor New York City has implemented a safety net protection policy: on the contrary, New York City Mayor Rudolph Giuliani seems more interested in privatizing the city's hospitals than in helping them survive in a managed care world.

What has changed, however, is the balance of power within the policymaking environment. Under the new regime, the influence of the commercial HMOs has increased substantially, while that of hospitals, unions, and advocates has declined, though it is too early to evaluate the extent or the permanence of the decline. The shifting politics is explained, in part, by national forces: the movement toward managed care is the dominant story of current U.S. health care policy. At the same time, the more conservative political environment makes it harder for the traditional groups to influence policy. Nonetheless, the policymaking environment remains extraordinarily fluid and uncertain.

The evolving policymaking environment will soon need to deal with several important substantive issues. There is, for example, real concern about the long-range viability of New York City's public hospital system. There are also questions about the quality of care provided by many of the managed care plans, few of whom are experienced in serving a low-income population. A recent state investigation concluded, for example, that many Medicaid beneficiaries have difficulty scheduling initial medical appointments.[37] Similarly, many beneficiaries are unable (or unwilling) to travel long distances to authorized providers. Others, without telephones, cannot follow treatment regimens that require telephone authorization. And still others cannot find authorized providers who speak their native languages. For all of these reasons, many enrollees still seek care in the public hospital emergency rooms.

This is not to suggest, of course, that all commercial HMOs are ill-equipped to treat the Medicaid population. But many have entered the market remarkably quickly, in the hope of capturing a large share of low-risk, low-cost Medicaid clients, and therefore have focused as much on marketing as on service. With many plans competing for clients (in some communities there are more than a dozen competitors), and with health plan marketing surprisingly deregulated, the potential for fraud is high. Indeed, state officials recently suspended direct marketing in New York City because of these concerns.[38]

Even with these problems, New York's Medicaid program is in the midst of a remarkable transition, moving steadily in the direction of managed care. Whether and how New York's Medicaid policymaking environment shifts as well is an important but still unanswerable question.

Medicaid Managed Care: Summary and Some Final Thoughts

In both California and New York there is serious competition now underway for the Medicaid business. This competition reverses (virtually overnight) the long-standing reluctance of commercial HMOs to court Medicaid clients. It also challenges the assumption that the managed care industry is too small to accommodate the Medicaid population. Moreover, the competition today is not (primarily) between newly formed fly-by-night organizations (as was the case in California during the early 1970s). Rather, several of the nation's largest HMOs (such as U.S. Healthcare and Oxford in New York and Blue Cross and Foundation Health in California) are pursuing vigorously the Medicaid client.[39]

Some observers attribute the newly competitive environment to the states' legislative activity, including the managed care initiatives themselves as well as the measures targeted directly at the HMO industry (such as the surcharge in New York and the threatened mandate in California). But while these actions surely had an impact, the competition in New York continued (even increased) after the courts voided the surcharge, and California's HMOs now seek to enroll far more than the hundred thousand Medi-Cal clients agreed on in the CAHMO Agreement.

As I noted earlier, the better explanation is that HMOs, initially pressured by government to enroll Medicaid beneficiaries, now recognize the wisdom of doing so. Medicaid clients (at least the low-risk, low-cost variety) generate profits. They also increase patient volume, which in turn increases negotiating leverage with hospitals and other providers.

The rapid expansion of Medicaid managed care can, if done well, improve the quality of care received by beneficiaries, encouraging more primary care and less emergency room use. There are, however, serious risks. First, it is unclear whether even the established HMOs have contracts with enough community-based providers (both physicians and others) to adequately serve their newly enrolled populations. This is especially true if Medicaid regulators can minimize adverse selection and compel the HMOs to take some of the sickest and most difficult to treat Medicaid clients (the babies addicted to cocaine, the AIDs victims, the mentally ill who are homeless).[40] But even the most attractive Medicaid clients (healthy women with young children) often need special attention: many neither speak English nor have a telephone, most have long used the local emergency room as their only provider, and nearly all live in medically underserved communities.

Second, the profitability of the Medicaid client may well diminish. For example, Medicaid officials try to reduce reimbursement rates whenever they conclude that a managed care organization is making excess profit. The San Mateo experience is illustrative: when the county-administered health insuring organization succeeded in keeping costs down and profits up, both federal and state officials insisted upon a rate reduction. Officials at New York's Bronx Health Plan report a similar pattern. Moreover, if Medicaid costs continue to soar, despite the emphasis on managed care (as they likely will), there will be additional pressure to lower HMO reimbursement rates. This is especially true in New York, where

HMOs receive from Medicaid between $140 and $160 per month per AFDC-related client (far more than their counterparts in California, who receive between $80 and $100 per month for each such client. Finally, if Medicaid officials ever reduce adverse selection, the profitability of the Medicaid client will diminish even further. As the profitability of Medicaid clients declines, so will their attractiveness to HMOs (particularly since the reform environment is now less threatening).

The lack of a long-term HMO commitment increases the need to preserve a strong medical safety net. California and New York have adopted very different approaches to the safety net protection issue. In California, state Medi-Cal officials have used their significant bureaucratic discretion to develop a managed care model (the "two-plan model") that is designed explicitly to protect safety net institutions. In New York, in contrast, state officials have neither designed nor implemented a safety net protection plan. Instead, the state delegated to its fifty-seven counties the task of designing and implementing the managed care initiative, and the safety net (particularly in New York City) fends for itself.

At the same time, the policymaking environments in both states are clearly evolving. In California, state officials have only recently exercised the bureaucratic discretion exercised regularly in other Medicaid policy arenas. Before 1992, Medi-Cal managed care policy was surprisingly pluralistic. Similarly, state officials in New York are (gingerly) seeking to exert increased bureaucratic discretion. While the policymaking environment is likely to remain pluralistic, the balance of power within that arena is surely changing. Nevertheless, the New York–California comparison suggests again that New York's Medicaid program is less regulatory than its reputation, while California's is hardly a model of free market competition. The comparison suggests also that states, despite their complaints of federal micromanagement, retain wide discretion to shape their Medicaid programs.

9

States and the U.S. Health Care System

The Importance of the Federalism Debate

For more than two hundred years, policymakers and policy analysts have struggled to determine an appropriate division of labor between the states and the federal government. Back in the eighteenth century, for example, the anti-federalists opposed the ratification of the United States Constitution on the ground that it vested too much authority in the central government. While the states' rights argument lost that early political battle, the Constitution itself hardly created a powerful federal government. To the contrary, until the 1930s, and the New Deal, the federal government remained relatively uninvolved in most domestic policy arenas.

Since the New Deal, however, the federal agenda has grown enormously, especially in the social welfare arena. There is now a federal safety net for those persons outside the labor force through no fault of their own (the so-called deserving poor). Medicaid is an important part of that safety net. As the federal safety net has grown, however, so too has the debate over the intergovernmental division of labor in the social welfare arena.

The history of Medicaid illustrates the point. Medicaid began in 1965 with an intergovernmental compromise between those who advocated national standards and those who preferred state discretion: the federal government set the general rules and the states adapted and implemented them. The intergovernmental balance of power then shifted several times. During the First Medicaid Era (from the mid-1960s to the mid-1980s) the states dominated: the result is wide interstate variation in every aspect of Medicaid policy.

By the mid-1980s, federal officials were ready to assert greater control. Congress required states to liberalize Medicaid eligibility criteria, expand medical benefit coverage, and increase provider reimbursement. Medicaid expenditures were soon rising rapidly. States responded by developing creative schemes to shift rising costs back to the federal treasury. The intergovernmental tension increased.

During the early 1990s, the tide turned again. The federal mandates were fewer, the waivers from federal law became more common, and many proposed converting Medicaid into a large block grant. The block grant proposal would provide states with a fixed sum of federal dollars with few strings and conditions. States would need to spend the money on health care for the poor but could decide whom to cover, what to cover, and how much to pay. Beneficiaries would no longer have a right to benefits. If there later is a perception that states are abusing this authority, the federal government could change its mind and add conditions and requirements. The intergovernmental battling would continue.

To some degree, the intergovernmental back-and-forth is inevitable: by vesting many of the same powers in separate governments the Constitution deliberately created much uncertainty and tension. Federalism is, after all, one of the checks and balances on government activity. There is a cost, however, and in the health care context the cost is significant. For this reason, the argument of this chapter is that the federal government needs to take a far more active role in shaping and structuring the U.S. health care system. Before making this argument, however, I begin with a brief history of American federalism. The history provides a context for how we got where we are. The history also suggests why the changes I propose will be difficult to achieve.

The Origins of American Federalism

Political institutions reflect political cultures, and American federalism is no exception. The origins of American federalism are found in two tenets of American political thought: first, that all people are endowed with certain inalienable rights (from the right to maintain private property to the right of free speech), and second, that government is a necessary evil needed primarily to protect the exercise of the individual rights.

During the Revolutionary War, there was a movement to strengthen America's national government. Some felt that to win the war the colonies needed a more centralized and powerful national administration. Others warned that the growing national debt required a federal taxing power. Still others claimed that only a strong central government could control the local mobs that took advantage of the chaos of war.

Despite these arguments, the movement to strengthen the national government met vigorous resistance. Why fight the British if victory would simply transfer power to another distant monarch? Instead, in 1781 the colonies enacted the Articles of Confederation, a "firm league of friendship" among the thirteen colonies. There would be a weak Congress (with members chosen by state legislatures), no president, and a limited national agenda.

Even after the war ended in 1783, the American settlers initially were uninterested in a strengthened national government. It took several years, in fact, before the Constitutional Convention was held in Philadelphia in 1787. And while some of the Founding Fathers (notably Alexander Hamilton) hoped to create a powerful national government, the debate was generally between those who wanted a large but relatively weak national government (such as James Madison) and those who wanted a small national government and powerful states (the anti-federalists).

Madison's defense of the Constitution is instructive.[1] He argued that individual rights are best protected in large republics because interest groups (or what he called "factions") can more easily dominate small governments. He added, however, that federal policymaking authority should be limited, that the exercise of such authority should be divided between three branches of government (legislative, executive, and judicial), and that each branch should act as a check and balance on the others. Moreover, all powers not delegated to the federal government are reserved to the states. The goal was to make federal action difficult to achieve.

The Evolution of Health Care Federalism

The bias against federal action dominated the first 150 years of U.S. politics. This bias was particularly strong in the social welfare context, where the tradition of the English poor laws remained strong. Social welfare programs were a local responsibility, and assistance was to be provided only to the "deserving poor." The main exception was the Civil War pension program, which provided federally administered benefits to Union veterans. More typical was President Franklin Pierce's decision, in 1854, to veto legislation granting federal land to states to develop hospitals for the mentally ill. According to Pierce, the legislation would unconstitutionally involve the federal government in a local welfare program.[2] Similarly, while the federal agenda expanded marginally during the Progressive Era (the early 1900s), the most influential progressives were Woodrow Wilson and the states' rights supporters, not Herbert Croly and the new nationalists.

For Franklin Roosevelt, however, politics as usual was a prescription for disaster — a decentralized and limited government simply could not effectively respond to an economic depression. Roosevelt envisioned, instead, a strong federal government, fueled by a power executive branch, in which economic and social welfare programs would be insulated from the localistic political process.

Roosevelt knew, however, that Congress was unwilling to establish a nationally administered social welfare system. The main obstacle were several southern Democrats who because of their long seniority chaired key congressional committees. The southerners worried that a national welfare system would undermine the southern sharecropper economy and provide too many benefits to children of former black slaves.[3] Roosevelt agreed to compromise, and the result was the bifurcated welfare system (that still exists today). The federal government finances and administers the popular "social insurance" programs (like Social Security), while the states administer, set policy for, and help finance the politically unpopular "welfare" programs (like AFDC).

The New Deal model of welfare federalism was challenged during the mid-1960s, an era in which President Lyndon B. Johnson proposed legislation to help turn the United States into a "Great Society." Johnson was influenced, of course, by the civil rights movement, which encouraged northern liberals to bypass state leaders wherever possible. Johnson was also influenced by a new cadre of social scientists who argued that poverty is caused primarily by social conditions (not by individual sloth) and that welfare programs should seek both to change those social conditions and to reduce the feelings of powerlessness and alienation that such conditions generated.

The new welfare federalism thus called for (some) federal funds to be dispersed directly to community-based groups (rather than through state or local politicians). Interestingly, however, the model was applied more consistently in the education, jobs, and welfare arenas than it was in the health care context. Federal funds were used, for example, to fund local Head Start programs (to give poor children a better chance to learn), job training programs (to provide the unemployed with useful skills), and day care programs (to provide mothers with needed child care). But while the community health center program followed the new welfare federalism model as well, the major health care initiatives of the day, Medicare and Medicaid, did not. These were classic New Deal-styled programs: the federal government finances and administers Medicare, while the states administer, set policy for, and help finance Medicaid.

The variation in health care federalism is related to variation in the goals of the health care programs. The community health center program was an effort to alter the nation's health care delivery system. The goal was to create community-run primary care clinics in indigent communities. The policy assumption was that poor people were too often receiving primary care services in the emergency rooms of large acute care hospitals. The plan was to enable poor people themselves to both create and administer the newly formed health centers.

Medicare and Medicaid, in contrast, were efforts to provide the aged and the poor with access to the existing mainstream health care system. They were medical insurance programs. They were not efforts to alter the existing health care delivery system. The legislative goal thus was to assure the influential medical community (especially the hospital industry) that the new programs would be generous and timely payers. Since poor people were to receive the same medical care as the middle class, there was no need for the poor to participate in the development of the program.

By the early 1970s, however, it was clear that Medicaid beneficiaries had not and would not obtain consistent and adequate access to the mainstream medical system. Medicaid reimbursement so favored institutional providers that only a small number of physicians were accepting Medicaid patients. Medicaid clients, like the uninsured, received health care mainly in the emergency rooms of large acute care hospitals.

Around this same time, however, the welfare federalism of the Great Society had come under attack. State and local officials complained vigorously that they were wrongly cut out of the policy loop. Academic researchers uncovered mismanagement and occasional fraud. Richard Nixon and his Republican advisors rejected the Great Society explanation for poverty. Nixon called for a "new federalism," under which power would return to state and local officials. While several Great Society programs continued to flourish (and remain with us today), the Great Society model of federalism was generally abandoned. The renewed emphasis on states' rights fit in well with the Medicaid intergovernmental balance of power: this was the era of state discretion and interstate variation.

U.S. federalism since the 1970s has emphasized states' rights. The political debate has generally assumed that federal officials have too much policymaking authority and states too little. Presidents from Nixon to Reagan to Clinton have proposed devolving power back to the states. Public support for states' rights remains strong. Nonetheless, the policy outcomes have not consistently reflected the rhetoric. During the Nixon era, for example, the federal agenda expanded significantly: not only did the federal government for the first time enact environmental protection and consumer protection laws, but Nixon himself proposed both national health insurance and national welfare reform. Similarly, while Reagan persuaded Congress to significantly cut federal aid to the states, Congress in the Reagan era was also responsible for the expanded federal regulation of Medicaid.

Since the 1994 congressional elections, however, the states' rights rhetoric has increased again, accompanied now by a Republican Congress that seems anxious to turn rhetoric into reality. Unlike earlier conservative eras, however, this time the states' rights supporters are joined, at least in the health care context, by a growing contingent of liberal reformers. The politics of federalism are becoming bipartisan.

The liberal argument for the states is straightforward. With the defeat of the various national health insurance proposals and the election of a conservative Republican Congress, the likelihood of national reform anytime soon is obviously slim (at best). There are, however, a handful of states that might implement major reform if only they had increased policymaking authority. If ERISA were amended, for example, some states might require employers to provide health insurance to their employees. Oregon is one such state. Other states might enact incremental insurance reforms. History even offers cause for optimism. As Richard Nathan argues, states are often most active in eras of federal retrenchment.[4]

The conservative argument for the states is equally straightforward: state policymaking arguably is more innovative, more democratic, and more pragmatic. There is a growing literature, for example, that suggests policy innovation is encouraged by decentralization and discouraged by centralization. This literature suggests that states can indeed be policy laboratories, trying and testing new and innovative policy options.

There also is wide support for the proposition that state and local politics is inherently more democratic than that which occurs in Washington, D.C. Citizens are supposedly more involved, politicians and bureaucrats are more accountable, and decisions are more responsive to local needs. This argument is especially relevant in health policy, since health care is an inherently local activity, revolving primarily around the relationship between provider and patient.

Finally, state politics is often considered more pragmatic and responsible. After all, most states are required by law to balance their budgets (in sharp contrast to the federal budget process). This budget discipline would, the argument goes, encourage state officials to enact and implement effective cost-containment procedures.

Health Care Federalism: Lessons From The California–New York Comparison

This book began with a question: Why does New York's Medicaid program cost so much more than California's? The case study that followed offered evidence on three important (and related) issues: interstate variation in a state-dominated health care program; bureaucratic discretion, and its influence on state policy; and the role states should play in a reformed health care system.

Interstate Variation

Policy analysts have written for years about the variation between southern welfare programs and those in the northeast. The programs in Alabama and Mississippi are typically compared with those in New York and New Jersey. The differences are great. The southern programs cover fewer persons, provide fewer benefits, and spend less money. The California–New York comparison demonstrates, however, that interstate variation is not limited to the usual suspects: the nation's two largest Medicaid programs, both with generous eligibility coverage and benefit packages, have produced substantially different spending patterns. Similarly situated states produce dissimilar programs.

The California–New York comparison also suggests that interstate variation exists in every facet of health care policy. Nursing home reimbursement in New York is more than double that provided in California. Home care coverage in New York is also more expansive and expensive. New York uses rate setting to reimburse hospitals, while California uses selective contracting. New York delegates responsibility for implementing managed care to the counties, while California keeps control in the state bureaucracy. And although both states provide a comparatively generous benefit package, California relies more heavily on prior authorization and utilization review than does New York.

The Bureaucratic Discretion Variable

As I noted earlier, there is an ongoing debate in political science over "who governs": who determines which programs are enacted, how such programs are implemented, and to whom power and resources are distributed? The traditional view is that U.S. politics is society-centered and group dominated. Policy is said to emerge incrementally, through negotiation and compromise between interested groups. Public officials are generally viewed as scorekeepers (enacting the consensus policy) or simply one of many key players.

The alternate view is that public officials are far more autonomous and influential than commonly supposed. Eric Nordlinger developed a three-prong typology to summarize the state-centered policy model.[5] First, there are occasions when state and societal preferences coincide. In these cases, public officials try to reinforce the consensus, thus forestalling future opposition. State officials might, for example, publicize the success of an ongoing program. Second, there are times when state and societal preferences initially conflict, but officials are able to persuade or defuse the opposition. Finally, public officials sometimes act autonomously despite vigorous opposition from key societal groups (though ongoing and overwhelming opposition causes even the most autonomous official to reconsider).

The debate between society-centered theorists and their state-centered counterparts suggests, in the words of Gabriel Almond, "a research program to distinguish among politics according to the degree to which state (governmental) personnel take the initiative in the making of public policy and the factors and conditions that explain these differences in degree."[6] Such an inquiry into federal health policymaking is now underway.

James Morone, for example, argues that federal health policy before 1970 was dominated by physicians (and their professional norms) and physician groups (primarily the American Medical Association).[7] In Morone's words, "legislators were solicitous, government bureaucrats deferential, patients obedient, payers passive."[8] As health care costs rose, however, pluralistic health care politics was replaced by bureaucratic politics. Doctors lost influence as health care administrators developed formula driven cost-containment initiatives. This change, notes Morone, has apparent advantages: programs appear to work scientifically (without politics), they are too complex to be turned into political symbols (seniors against DRGs isn't catchy), and they are quite narrow (and thus feasible). The disadvantage is that physicians have lost authority, and the system has lost accountability.

Lawrence Brown agrees that federal health politics between 1945 and 1970 was pluralistic (though physicians occupy a less dominant place in his description of the interest-group tussles).[9] He also agrees that federal health politics since then has been decidedly state-centered (though he suggests that policymakers look for help to nongovernmental policy analysts more than to the public bureaucracy). He even suggests that Clinton's health reform effort failed, in part, because of a backlash against the policy analysts (long quiescent groups rejected the effort to have technical experts redo the entire U.S. health care system).[10]

Along with the macro analyses provided by Morone and Brown, other political scientists provide in-depth descriptions of governance battles in particular federal programs or institutions. Thomas Oliver, for example, describes in great detail how bureaucratic experts (in the federal Physician Payment Review Commission) persuaded Congress to institute a new Medicare physician payment methodology.[11] Mark Peterson offers a similarly detailed description of congressional health care politics.[12]

There are far fewer efforts, however, to study the governance of federal-state health care programs (like Medicaid), or state health care policy more generally. To what degree is state health care politics society-centered? To what extent do state bureaucrats influence policy (either through the legislative process or through the implementation of enacted laws)? Who governs?

Robert Hackey considers these issues in his comparison of hospital reimbursement policy in four states (New York, Massachusetts, New Hampshire, and Rhode Island).[13] Hackey suggests that state health policies differ, at least in part, because state health bureaucrats operate in different political regimes: in imposed regimes, bureaucrats have significant discretion and can enforce strict cost-containment initiatives; in negotiated regimes, bureaucrats negotiate and bargain with powerful interest groups; and in market regimes, bureaucratic influence is minimal and societal groups dominate. Hackey's model is powerful and useful (though I disagree with his conclusion that bureaucrats in New York operate in an imposed regime). Other than Hackey, however, the literature on state health governance is surprisingly thin. Similarly, other than Malcolm Goggin's study of Medicaid child health programs,[14] the literature on intergovernmental health governance is equally thin.

One goal of this book is to join the debate over health care governance. Who governs the Medicaid programs in California and New York? Why does New York spend so much more than California? What explains the interstate variation in Medicaid?

The study suggests that variation in Medicaid spending is due in large part to variation in bureaucratic discretion. California officials have significant discretion to implement a cost-control agenda. The broad discretion is rooted in three variables. First, California's administrative agencies are unusually insulated from legislative tinkering. Hospital reimbursement policy illustrates the point. The California Medical Assistance Commission sets reimbursement rates without interference from the state legislature. This differs substantially from New York, where the legislature regularly resolves reimbursement disputes. Second, executive branch leaders (from Ronald Reagan to Pete Wilson) have consistently emphasized the cost-control mission. The organizational goals are thus clear. Third, many important interest groups (hospitals, health care unions, and consumer advocates) are relatively weak; others (nursing homes) accept the cost-control bargain (low rates coupled with minimal quality oversight).

The bureaucracy in New York operates in a very different political environment. Medicaid politics in New York is fragmented, decentralized, and pluralistic. Provider groups, labor leaders, and consumer advocates all exercise significant policy authority. So too do local officials, bureaucrats in a host of state agencies, and legislative leaders. At the same time, executive branch leaders (from Rockefeller to Cuomo) have had an evolving list of priorities, leaving Medicaid bureaucrats without a strong organizational identity. The result is high costs, particularly in the long-term care policy arena.

To be sure, neither state presents a pure policymaking model. Interest groups in California were once quite influential in developing managed care policy, and hope to reassert their authority in the future. Conversely, New York State regulators sometimes act autonomously (especially in budget crises). At the same time, federal officials are pressuring California to regulate more closely the quality of care provided in nursing homes. Meanwhile, budget constraints lead New York policymakers to consider reductions in home health care services. In both states, however, there is resistance to change. California's reluctance to implement the nursing home quality-of-care regulations imposed by Congress is illustrative. So too is New York's unwillingness to more stringently restrict the availability of round-the-clock home health care. The result (in both states) is a series of incremental adjustments: Medi-Cal will implement (grudgingly) the nursing home reforms, and New York will (minimally) restrict the availability of home care services.

There is a pattern that seems to be at work: a state's political history produces a particular policymaking environment; the policymaking environment encourages particular policy choices; and both the policymaking environment and the policy choices are difficult to alter. There is also a lesson: the pluralist versus state-centered debate depends, in part, on the policy and the state examined.

States (and the Limits of State Health Policy)

There is strong political support for delegating increased policymaking authority to the states. Medicaid and AFDC may well be converted into block grants. At a minimum, state flexibility and discretion under the programs is likely to increase. One justification for the trend is that states (and their political subdivisions) act as policy laboratories, developing and testing innovative programs, replicating initiatives that work and abandoning those that do not. This argument is not without merit. This book even illustrates one way in which states can be laboratories.

The hypothesis generated by the California–New York comparison (that bureaucratic centralization influences Medicaid spending patterns) is testable and generalizable. Researchers could, for example, examine the relationship between bureaucratic centralization and Medicaid spending in other states.

Similarly, both New York and California are now testing

grounds for a host of innovative policy ideas. Some of these innovations were described at length earlier. Medicaid managed care is
one. Cluster care home care services are another. Reimbursement
systems are a third (selective contracting in California versus rate
setting in New York).

Other innovations are being tested as well. Both states, for example, are experimenting with a new model for financing long-
term care under which public and private payers share the costs
and risks. This "public-private" model encourages consumers to
buy two or three years of private nursing home insurance by permitting them to become Medicaid-eligible when the fixed term
expires, without having to exhaust or transfer their assets. The
initiative appeals to insurers (who tap a new market) and Medicaid officials (who hope to save money), and it is now being implemented in New York, California, Connecticut, and Indiana. The
(presumably contrasting) records of the states could shed light on
how to design, market, price, administer, and refine these new
insurance products.

Another demonstration project builds on a small but impressive
program in San Francisco, called On-Lok, which serves aged and
indigent individuals, all of whom are eligible for placement in
skilled nursing facilities but instead live at home, attend a day
treatment center, and get care from On-Lok workers. Medicaid
and Medicare give On-Lok a fixed fee for each client; in exchange,
it bears full responsibility for the clients' care. By most accounts,
On-Lok is a successful, cost-effective, and high-quality program
and one of the few efforts to manage the care of the aged and
indigent. Congress, hoping to test whether the model should be
expanded, has now authorized a dozen replication sites around the
country, including two in New York (one in the Bronx and one in
Rochester).

Policy analysts (including this one) work hard to evaluate these
programs and to suggest lessons learned. Oftentimes, the recom-
mendation is to replicate the innovative activity. Several analysts,
for example, documented the success of state hospital rate-setting

initiatives and recommended the replication of the model. There is surprisingly little evidence, however, that states import policies first implemented elsewhere. Most states, for example, debated the merits of hospital rate setting, but only a handful found it appealing enough to adopt and retain. Nearly every state is experimenting with Medicaid managed care, but the managed care programs now being implemented are highly diverse. And although Oregon drew national attention when it adopted a "health care rationing" experiment, no state has followed suit.

The problem, once again, is that it is difficult for state policymakers to escape their state-based political environments. States instead look curiously at approaches taken in other states but then adopt initiatives that reflect state politics. This finding is illustrated by the comparison of Medicaid managed care in California and New York. Both states have established expanded managed care enrollment as a high priority. But the previous policymaking environment shapes the current managed care initiative: New York's effort is decentralized and pluralistic; California's is more state-centered. Similarly, fee-for-service Medicaid in New York is unusually costly, and managed care rates now in place reflect those patterns. Conversely, fee-for-service Medicaid in California is unusually low and its managed care payment levels are also low.

This outcome is not necessarily bad. Interstate variation is not always inappropriate. Some even suggest that state discretion and the resultant policy variation reflect the values of democratic governance and local responsiveness: health policy established at the state level is presumably more democratic and more responsive than policy established by bureaucrats in the nation's capitol. But does the evidence support this claim? Are state governments more democratic or more responsive than their federal counterpart?

Consider four criteria for democratic activity: participation, trust, knowledge, and accountability. Start with participation. There is a cadre of citizens who participate in local planning commissions, town school boards, and other institutions of local government. Citizens do not, however, participate to the same degree in institutions of state (or national) government. At the same time, there is little evidence that citizens trust state officials any more than they trust their federal counterparts. For example, every year from 1972 to 1991 the U.S. Advisory Commission on Intergovernmental Relations asked the question "from which level of government do you feel you get the most for your money?" Eleven times the federal government ranked first, seven times local government did, and one time the two levels tied for first. State government ranked last eighteen times.[15]

Finally, what about knowledge and accountability? Most people are far more knowledgeable about national issues than state and could name their congressman but not their state senator. This wouldn't matter if state officials were more accountable than their federal counterparts. But there is not any evidence that supports this proposition either.

In any event, issues of democracy and accountability become particularly murky in the context of most health care policy. Consider health care financing, the subject of much of this book. Health care financing in California and New York is hardly textbook democracy. In California, decisions are made by autonomous bureaucrats. In New York, the decision-making process seems more open, but few citizens are themselves aware or involved. In neither state is the process especially democratic (though bureaucrats in both states are accountable ultimately to elected officials). Nonetheless, democratic decision-making may not be the best way to develop reimbursement policy. Government (at any level) seeks to be a prudent purchaser: accountability comes primarily from the financial bottom line, not from public participation. Indeed, one lesson of the California–New York comparison is that cost containment may require bureaucratic centralization not interest-group politics.

Medicaid eligibility policy, in contrast, does seem to be relatively democratic, at least if we define democratic outcomes as those produced by the state legislative process. Medicaid eligibility criteria is set by legislators, not bureaucrats. This democratic process has, however, produced wide interstate variation in coverage. Here democratic decision making may clash with other important values, in this case the principle that access to health care should not depend on place of residence. Government should guarantee access to care; medical coverage should not be decided at the ballot box. No person should die because they are unable to afford medical care.

Universal insurance is justified, of course, not just on philosophical grounds but on pragmatic grounds as well. The uninsured receive health care, especially in emergency situations, but often cannot pay the cost of the care. This leads medical providers, especially hospitals, to shift the cost of caring for the uninsured onto other payers, especially private insurers. This practice leads private insurers to raise premiums (to pay for the increased pay outs) and to market their product more selectively, denying coverage to high-risk individuals (such as persons with preexisting medical conditions or persons employed in high-risk occupations). These practices raise the nation's health care bill even further and simultaneously increase the number of the uninsured, which begins the cost-shifting cycle yet again.

States by themselves, however, will not implement universal insurance programs. One obstacle is money: coverage for uninsured persons is expensive. States are restrained also by the fear of business exodus: the interstate competition for business drives states to reduce taxes and regulations, and insurance reforms generally require more of both. Then there are federal laws that explicitly limit state reform activities. ERISA, for example, prevents states from imposing employer mandates and from regulating or taxing companies that self-insure. Finally, even were Congress to remove the ERISA obstacle (which seems unlikely), few states seem likely to summon the political will to actually implement comprehensive reform. This is especially true since states' ability to control health care costs is limited, and insurance reform without effective cost controls is a recipe for disaster. As Deborah Stone has pointed out, "it is impossible to regulate the health care system effectively if you can only regulate a part of it."[16]

This suggests the need to rethink the division of labor in the health policy arena.[17] Certain decisions need to be made on a national level. First is a federal mandate of universal health insurance. Second is a minimum benefit package. Third is a financing framework. Such a framework requires both a way of raising money (whether through special taxes, employer premiums, or general revenues) and a way of containing costs (whether through global budgets, premium caps, or market-based strategies). Other decisions should be made on a state or local level. Capital planning is an obvious example. Regulating medical education and licensure is another. Public health is a third.

One model for reform would be to expand the Medicare program. Here is a popular and well-run social insurance program that has worked well for more than thirty years and that has developed and implemented innovative cost-containment strategies (in both the hospital and physician reimbursement arena). Here also is a program with clear lines of accountability (there is no complicated intergovernmental division of labor) and low administrative costs. Medicare could even be expanded to cover only the uninsured and the Medicaid populations, leaving intact the existing private health insurance industry. Under this approach, the successful Medicare reimbursement systems could be imposed on all payers. A second and more radical option is to make Medicare the single payer for the entire health care system. Under either scenario, however, universal coverage would be achieved and overall health care costs controlled.[18]

A third option for reform, less nationalist in scope, is for the federal government to establish a menu of choices for reform and to supervise state implementation of those reforms. Congress could, for example, offer states three reform frameworks: managed competition with an employer mandate, a state-run single-payer system financed primarily by an increased payroll tax, or an expanded

Medicare program. Congress could also offer three or four benefit coverage packages. Under a menu system, the federal government would make the toughest political choices (such as universal coverage), but states could become true policy laboratories, trying and testing different approaches in a relatively controlled environment. Over time, for example, researchers could examine, evaluate, and compare the successes or failures of the models. Which model best controls costs? Which encourages good quality care? Which produces the highest consumer satisfaction? Is one of the models suited for nationwide replication, or should states maintain indefinitely the ability to choose?

A fourth option is the Canadian model. Under that intergovernmental partnership, the ten Canadian provinces tailor the health care system to local needs while meeting five national criteria: the programs must provide universal, comprehensive, accessible, portable, and publicly administered coverage. The national government, by setting forth governing principles, ensures that all citizens receive comprehensive and accessible health care. The provinces, meanwhile, by establishing their own programs, ensure that the system is responsive to local conditions.[19]

This is obviously a very rough sketch of four very broad options. The point is, however, that certain decisions about the health care system need to be made nationally. The federal government needs to manage health care federalism. Managing federalism along these lines does not imply bypassing the states; it does suggest, however, that the current emphasis on increased state authority is misguided.

To be sure, there is little likelihood that Congress will enact national health insurance anytime soon. There is even less likelihood that Medicare will be the basis for a national reform initiative. Even during last year's health reform debate, when national health insurance for a time seemed likely, Medicare was never the model of choice. Instead, nearly all reform proposals (with the exception of Congressman Pete Stark's) delegated key policymaking and administrative tasks to the states.

Indeed, rather than expanding Medicare, the current Congress seems intent on cutting the programs funding. But while the proposals to cut Medicare spending are portrayed as efforts to save the program from impending bankruptcy (since the programs current mix of taxes and premiums is inadequate to cover program costs), the initiatives are motivated primarily by the desire to balance the federal budget (while also implementing a tax cut).

The coming cuts in the Medicare and Medicaid programs will lead inevitably to a worsened health care crisis. The number of uninsured will rise. The cost shifting in the system will increase. Overall costs will continue to rise. Eventually, health care reform will return to the national agenda. When it does, reformers should propose a nationally managed federalism, under which the federal government establishes the framework for reform. U.S. history suggests that enacting such a proposal will be difficult. The American bias in favor of state-based reforms is strong. But without a federal policy framework the nation's health care crisis will only get worse.

Notes

Chapter 1

1. Mathematica Policy Research, *Managed Care and Low Income Populations: A Case Study of Managed Care in Tennessee* (Washington, D.C.: The Henry J. Kaiser Foundation and the Commonwealth Fund, 1995).

2. Mathematica Policy Research, *Managed Care and Low Income Populations: A Case Study of Managed Care in Oregon* (Washington, D.C.: The Henry J. Kaiser Foundation and the Commonwealth Fund, 1995).

3. Deane Neubauer, "Hawaii: A Pioneer in Health Systems Reform," *Health Affairs* vol. 12, no. 2 (Summer 1993), pp. 31–39.

4. Mathematica Policy Research, *Managed Care and Low Income Populations: A Case Study of Managed Care in Minnesota* (Washington, D.C.: The Henry J. Kaiser Foundation and the Commonwealth Fund, 1995).

5. Robert A. Crittenden, "Managed Competition and Premium Caps in Washington State," *Health Affairs* vol. 12, no. 2 (Summer 1993), pp. 82–88.

6. The National Commission on the State and Local Public Service, *Frustrated Federalism: Rx for State and Local Health Care Reform* (Albany: Rockefeller Institute of Government, 1993).

7. The differences between the two groups are also clear. Liberals, for example, generally oppose both the movement toward block grants and the effort to dramatically cut federal health and welfare spending.

8. Dick Nathan, the Director of the Rockefeller Institute, in Albany, NY, coined the term "devolution revolution."

9. One such organization is the Intergovernmental Health Policy Project, which is affiliated with George Washington University. Another is the Alpha Center in Washington, D.C.

10. A good example is *Five States That Could Not Wait: Lessons For Health Reform From Florida, Hawaii, Minnesota, Oregon, and Vermont,* eds. Daniel M. Fox and John K. Iglehart (Cambridge, MA: Blackwell Publishers, 1994). Another book on state leaders is *Health Policy Reform in America: Innovations from the States,* ed. Howard M. Leichter (Armonk, NY: M.E. Sharpe, 1992).

11. 29 U.S.C. sections 1001–1461 (Supp. IV 1992).

12. In 1974, Hawaii enacted a requirement that employers provide their employees with health insurance. Shortly thereafter, the federal courts held that Hawaii's mandate violated ERISA. *Standard Oil Company v. Agsalud,* 633 F. 2d 760

(9th Cir. 1980), *aff'd,* 454 U.S. 801 (1981). In 1983, after a difficult legislative battle, Congress granted the state an ERISA waiver, largely because the mandate was enacted before ERISA itself was passed. Since that time, however, Congress has not only rejected waiver applications from numerous mainland states, it has also rejected Hawaii's application to alter the terms of its waiver.

13. Diane Rowland, "Health Care of the Poor: The Contribution of Social Insurance," in *Medical Care and the Health of the Poor,* eds. David E. Rogers and Eli Ginzberg (Boulder, CO: Westview Press, 1993), pp. 107–124.

14. Congressional Research Service, *Medicaid Source Book,* Tables III-1 and III-6, pp. 172, 194.

15. Prospective Payment Assessment Commission, *Medicare and the American Health Care System: Report to Congress* (Washington, D.C.: Prospective Payment Assessment Commission, June 1993), Table 5-14, p. 133.

16. General Accounting Office, "Medicaid: Spending Pressures Drive States toward Program Reinvention," *GAO/HEHS-95-122* (April 1995), Table 1.1, p. 18.

17. This phrase is borrowed from Robert Dahl's important study of politics in New Haven, *Who Governs?* (Chicago: University of Chicago Press, 1954).

18. Ibid.

19. E.E. Schattschneider, *The Semi-Sovereign People* (New York: Holt, Rinehart and Winston, 1960); Kay Lehman Schlozman and John T. Tierney, *Organized Interests and American Democracy* (New York: Harper & Row, 1986).

20. Eric Nordlinger, *On the Autonomy of the Democratic State* (Cambridge, MA: Harvard University Press, 1981).

Chapter 2

1. While Franklin Roosevelt supported national health insurance, he downplayed the issue early on, fearing a backlash that could undermine his entire New Deal agenda. Theodore Marmor, *The Politics of Medicare* (New York: Aldine Publishing Co., 1973), p. 9.

2. The best history of these efforts is contained in Paul Starr, *The Transformation of American Medicine* (New York: Basic Books, 1982).

3. The *Hospital Survey and Construction Act of 1946* (generally referred to as the *Hill-Burton Act*).

4. I borrow the term "welfare medicine" from an early history of the Medicaid program, by Robert Stevens and Rosemary Stevens, entitled *Welfare Medicine in America: A Case Study of Medicaid* (New York: The Free Press, 1974).

5. Theodore Marmor, *The Politics of Medicare* (New York: Aldine Publishing Co., 1973), p. 37.

6. The federal government does delegate many administrative tasks, such as processing payment claims, to private insurance carriers.

7. America's first private insurance companies, the Blue Cross systems that began during the 1930s, were often established by groups of hospitals in an effort to ensure that patients could pay their hospital bills. The long-standing relationship between hospitals and insurers helps explain why hospital reimbursement systems have long been generous.

8. Suzanne W. Letsch, "National Health Spending in 1991," *Health Affairs* (Spring 1993), p. 97.

9. Ibid., p. 96.

10. Karen Davis and Cathy Schoen, *Health and the War on Poverty* (Washington, D.C.: Brookings Institution, 1978).

11. General Accounting Office, "Community Health Centers: Challenges in Transitioning to Prepaid Managed Care," *GAO/HEHS-95-138* (May 1995), p. 1.

12. David S. Abernathy and David A. Pearson, *Regulating Hospital Costs: The Development of Public Policy* (Washington, D.C. and Ann Arbor: AUPHA Press, 1979).

13. Lawrence D. Brown, "Knowledge and Power: Health Services Research as a Political Resource," in E. Ginzberg (ed.), *Health Services Research: Key to Health Policy* (Cambridge: Harvard University Press, 1991).

14. Ibid.

15. Ibid. at 23.

16. Jon Oberlander, "Medicare and National Health Insurance: The Road Not Taken," a paper delivered at the 1994 Annual Meeting of the American Political Science Association, New York City, September 1 to September 4, 1994.

17. Prospective Payment Assessment Commission, *Medicare and the American Health Care System: Report to Congress* (Washington, D.C.: Prospective Payment Assessment Commission, June 1995), Table 5-15, p. 134.

18. There are a multitude of institutional arrangements that today go under the rubric of "managed care," including a variety of health maintenance organization (HMO) models, in which the HMO gets a fixed fee for each participant, regardless of his or her actual medical costs; preferred provider organizations (PPOs), in which a network of providers cares for an insured group in exchange for a (reduced) fee-for-service; and point-of-service organizations (POSs), in which consumers have a fiscal incentive to use in-network physicians but can, for a higher fee, see other providers as well. For a good description of these and other managed care hybrids, see Jonathan P. Weiner and Gregory de Lissovoy, "Razing a Tower of Babel: A Taxonomy for Managed Care and Health Insurance Plans," *Journal of Health Politics, Policy and Law,* vol. 18 (1993), pp. 75–103.

19. Prospective Payment Assessment Commission, *Medicare and the American Health Care System: Report to Congress* (June 1995), Table 5-16, p. 136.

20. There is evidence that staff model HMOs, in which clients receive their care from salaried HMO employees, do decrease health care costs. But much of the

managed care growth is in less restrictive organizations, such as independent practice associations, in which the HMO signs contracts with various independent
practitioners, and consumers choose from among the participating providers.
There is no hard evidence that arrangements like these encourage significant cost
savings. For a good review of the literature, see Linda J. Blumberg, "Managed Care
and Its Implications for Managed Competition," a report issued in April 1993 by
the Urban Institute.

21. Moreover, during this period Congress actually required states to expand
their coverage of certain groups, particularly pregnant women and children.

22. The Kaiser Commission on the Future of Medicaid, *Medicaid and Managed
Care: Lessons from the Literature* (Washington, DC: Kaiser Commission on the
Future of Medicaid, 1995).

23. The *McCarran-Ferguson Act* states: "the business of insurance . . . shall be
subject to the laws of the several States which relate to the regulation or taxation of
such business." 15 U.S.C. section 1012(a) (1988 and Supp. IV 1993). However,
federal laws, such as ERISA, that immunize self-insured companies from state
regulation may preempt state law. For a helpful description of the variation in state
regulatory activities, see General Accounting Office, "Health Insurance Regulation: Wide Variation in States' Authority, Oversight, and Resources," *GAO/
HRD-94-26* (1994).

24. State officials license and supervise physicians, nurses, and other health
professionals. While the licensing and certification process varies widely, every state
imposes minimum quality-of-care requirements. See generally, Prospective Payment Assessment Commission, *Medicare and the American Health Care System:
Report to Congress* (Washington, D.C.: Prospective Payment Assessment Commission, June 1993), p. 148.

25. In 1991, state and local governments paid 14.2 percent of the nation's $752
billion health care bill. Susan W. Letsch, Helen C. Lazenby, Katherine R. Levit, and
Cathy Cowan, "National Health Expenditures," *Health Care Financing Review*
(Winter 1992), pp. 14, 18.

26. *New State Ice Co. v. Liebmann,* 285 U.S. 262, 311 (1932) (Brandeis, J.,
dissenting).

27. See generally, Frank J. Thompson, "New Federalism and Health Care Policy: States and the Old Questions," *Journal of Health Politics, Policy and Law* vol. 11
(1986), p. 647.

28. Jill Quadagno, "From Old-Age Assistance to Supplemental Security In-
come: The Political Economy of Relief in the South, 1935–1972," in *The Politics of
Social Policy in the United States,* eds. Margaret Weir, Ann Shola Orloff, and Theda
Skocpol (Princeton, NJ: Princeton University Press, 1988), pp. 235–279.

29. James T. Patterson, *The New Deal and the States* (Westport: Greenwood
Press, 1969), p. 325.

30. Paul Peterson, Barry G. Rabe and Kenneth K. Wong, *When Federalism Works* (Washington, D.C.: Brookings Institution, 1986).

31. The Second Report of the National Commission on the State and Local Public Service, *Frustrated Federalism: Rx for State and Local Health Care Reform* (Albany: Rockefeller Institute of Government, 1993), p. 15.

32. For a good discussion of the implementation issues raised by the proposed health alliances, see James R. Tallon Jr. and Lawrence D. Brown, "Health Alliances: Functions, Forms and Federalism," in *Making Health Reform Work: The View from the States,* eds. John J. DiIulio Jr. and Richard P. Nathan (Washington, D.C.: Brookings Institution, 1994).

33. Robert G. Evans, "Canada: The Real Issues," *Journal of Health Politics, Policy and Law* vol. 17 (1992), pp. 739, 742–743.

34. The *Times* editorial page was an enthusiastic supporter of managed competition.

35. The architects of the Clinton plan assumed that the subsidies to be provided to small business to help fund the cost of the insurance provided would reduce small business opposition to the plan. It didn't.

36. The plan would, for example, have provided the aged with an expanded prescription drug benefit.

37. The purpose of this proposal was to increase the number of generalist physicians and reduce the oversupply of specialists. For a discussion of this initiative, see Michael S. Sparer, "Reform the Medical Workforce: Options and Opportunities," in *Making Health Reform Work: The View from the States,* eds. John J. DiIulio Jr. and Richard P. Nathan (Washington, D.C.: Brookings Institution, 1994).

38. Newt Gingrich, the first Republican Speaker of the House in forty years, is clearly trying to reassert the power of the congressional leadership. Whether he succeeds, and for how long, is still to be determined.

39. Former President George Bush received 38 percent of the vote and third-party candidate H. Ross Perot received 19 percent.

Chapter 3

1. John Holahan, Diane Rowland, Judith Feder, and David Heslam, "Explaining the Recent Growth in Medicaid Spending," *Health Affairs* vol. 12, no. 3 (Fall 1993), p. 177.

2. The 1987 and 1991 figures are from Jeffrey A. Buck and John Klemm, "Recent Trends in Medicaid Expenditures," *Health Care Financing Review: 1992 Annual Supplement* (Baltimore: U.S. Department of Health and Human Services, 1993), Table 13.6, p. 277. The 1993 data are from the General Accounting Office, "Medicaid: Restructuring Approaches Leave Many Questions," *GAO/HEHS-95-103* (April, 1995), Appendix 1, pp. 20–21.

3. GAO Report (note 2).

4. The National Commission on the State and Local Public Service, *Frustrated Federalism: Rx for State and Local Health Care Reform* (Albany: Rockefeller Institute of Government, 1993), p. 15.

5. 42 U.S.C. 1396a(a) *et seq.*

6. In 1965, in the early days of the Medicaid program, federal officials seemed poised to impose stringent national standards on all states participating in the program. Congress required, for example, that by July 1, 1975, states needed to ensure that "substantially all" recipients received "comprehensive care and services" (Section 1903[e] of the original Medicaid statute). This provision required states to do more than pay medical bills: states also had to develop plans and systems to ensure that recipients actually received comprehensive and high quality care. By the late 1960s, however, Medicaid costs were significantly higher than expected, and Congress was retreating rapidly from its ambitious agenda. In 1969, for example, Congress postponed the effective date of the "comprehensive care" requirement until 1977, and in 1972 it repealed the requirement altogether.

7. See Section 209(b) of the *Social Security Act Amendments of 1972.*

8. Congressional Research Service, *Medicaid Source Book,* Table III-9, p. 204.

9. Generally speaking, persons are categorically eligible for cash assistance if they are aged, blind, disabled, or in single-parent families. Even if categorically eligible, however, persons cannot receive welfare unless their income is below income eligibility levels.

10. Congressional Research Service, *Medicaid Source Book,* Table III-6, p. 194, sets forth the states with such programs.

11. Ibid. Federal law does require, however, that the Medicaid income level not exceed 133.3 percent of the state's AFDC income eligibility level.

12. 42 C.F.R. 435.301.

13. Congressional Research Service, *Medicaid Source Book,* p. 268. States cannot, however, impose such limits on infants or children under age six receiving care in certain safety-net hospitals.

14. Ibid. Table IV-3, pp. 269–274.

15. Ibid. Table IV-4, pp. 276–282.

16. Ibid. Table IV-6, pp. 286–289.

17. 42 C.F.R. 440.230(c).

18. See, for example, *Charleston Memorial Hospital v. Conrad,* 693 F. 2d 324 (4th Cir. 1982), (twelve day cap on inpatient hospital care imposed by South Carolina is reasonable); *Virginia Hospital Assn. v. Kenley,* 427 F. Supp. 781 (E.D. Va. 1977), (twenty-one day cap on inpatient hospital care imposed by Virginia is reasonable); and *Curtis v. Taylor,* 625 F. 2d 645 (5th Cir. 1980), (three visit per month cap on physician visits is reasonable).

19. Prospective Payment Assessment Commission, *Medicare and the American*

Health Care System (Washington, D.C.: Prospective Payment Assessment Commission, June 1995), Tables 5-14 and 5-15, pp. 133–134. Hospitals made up for their losses in Medicaid and Medicare by increasing charges to private insurers. For that reason, private insurers paid 129 percent of their clients' actual costs.

20. In 1994, for example, Medicare paid physicians approximately 64 percent of the average private insurance rate. Physician Payment Review Commission, *Annual Report to Congress: 1995* (Washington, D.C.: Physician Payment Review Commission, 1995), p. 76. In 1989 (the most recent year for which data is available), Medicaid paid physicians approximately 64 percent of the average Medicare rate. Physician Payment Review Commission, *Annual Report to Congress: 1993* (Washington, D.C.: Physician Payment Review Commission, 1993), p. 139.

21. *Conn. State Dept. of Public Welfare v. HEW,* 448 F. 2d 209 (2d Cir. 1971).

22. 45 C.F.R. 250.30(b); 42 U.S.C. 1396a(a) (13) (D).

23. *California Hospital Ass'n v. Obledo,* 602 F. 2d 1357 (9th Cir. 1979).

24. See, for example, *Mass. General Hospital v. Weiner,* 569 F. 2d 1156 (1st Cir. 1978); *New York City Health and Hospitals Corp. v. Blum,* 708 F. 2d 880 (2d Cir. 1983); and *Hempstead Gen. Hosp. v. Whalen,* 474 F. Supp. 398 (E.D.N.Y. 1979), *aff'd w/o published opinion,* 622 F. 2d 573 (2d Cir. 1977).

25. John Holahan and Joel W. Cohen, *Medicaid: The Trade-Off between Cost Containment and Access to Care* (Washington, D.C.: Urban Institute Press, 1986), p. 56.

26. Bruce Vladeck, *Unloving Care: The Nursing Home Tragedy* (New York: Basic Books, 1980), p. 52.

27. Chapter Five discusses why the variation in nursing home reimbursement between New York and California was (and still is) so extreme.

28. *Briarcliff Haven v. Dept. of Hum. Res.,* 403 F. Supp. 1355 (N.D. Ga. 1975).

29. Sanford L. Weiner and Susan S. Lehrer, *The Afterthought Industry: Developing Reimbursement Policy for Nursing Homes* (Unpublished report, 1980), pp. 8–10.

30. Ibid., p. 9.

31. See, for example, *Alabama Nursing Home Ass'n v. Califano,* 433 F. Supp. 1325 (M.D. Ala. 1977), and *Golden Isles Convalescent Ctr. v. Califano,* 442 F. Supp. 201 (S.D. Fla. 1977).

32. *Florida Dept. of Health and Rehabilitative Services v. Florida Nursing Home Ass'n,* 101 S. Ct. 1032 (1981).

33. 42 U.S.C. 1396a(a) (13) (A).

34. Physician Payment Review Commission, *Annual Report to Congress: 1994* (Washington, D.C.: Physician Payment Review Commission, 1994), Table 18-4, p. 356.

35. Thomas Fanning and Martin de Alteriis, "The Limits of Marginal Incentives in the Medicaid Program: Concerns and Cautions," *Journal of Health Politics, Policy and Law* vol. 18, no. 1 (Spring 1993), p. 29.

36. Teresa A. Coughlin, Leighton Ku, and John Holahan, *Medicaid since 1980: Costs, Coverage, and the Shifting Alliance between the Federal Government and the States* (Washington, D.C.: Urban Institute Press, 1994), p. 65.

37. Ibid., Table 3.1, p. 37.

38. Congressional Research Service, *Medicaid Source Book,* p. 35.

39. The increased enrollment is attributable to other factors also. The economic recession during the late 1980s contributed to program growth, as did the arrival of new epidemics, such as AIDS. John Holahan et al., "Explaining the Recent Growth in Medicaid Spending," p. 185.

40. Teresa A. Coughlin, Leighton Ku, and John Holahan, *Medicaid since 1980: Costs, Coverage, and the Shifting Alliance between the Federal Government and the States* (Washington, D.C.: Urban Institute Press, 1994), p. 139.

41. 42 U.S.C. sections 1395i-3(a)–(h) and 42 U.S.C. sections 1396r(a)–(h).

42. 42 U.S.C. section 1396a(a) (13) (A).

43. Ibid.

44. By 1989, for example, only three states still paid for nursing home care retrospectively, based on actual bills submitted. Congressional Research Service, *Medicaid Source Book,* p. 335.

45. 42 U.S.C. 1396a(a) (13) (A).

46. John Holahan and Joel Cohen, *Medicaid: The Trade-Off between Cost Containment and Access to Care* (Washington, D.C.: The Urban Institute Press, 1986), p. 57.

47. Congressional Research Service, *Medicaid Source Book,* p. 310.

48. Table V-1 of the *Medicaid Source Book,* found at pages 311–315, lists all the states and the inpatient payment methodologies they adopted.

49. In 1983, Congress changed the formula by which Medicare reimbursed hospitals, abandoning the actual cost approach and adopting in its stead a DRG system.

50. See also, *Colorado Health Care v. Colorado Dept. of Social Services,* 842 F. 2d 1158 (10th Cir. 1988); *Wisconsin Hosp. Ass'n v. Reivitz,* 733 F. 2d 1226 (7th Cir. 1984); and *Carbon Hill Health Care v. Beasley,* 528 F. Supp. 421 (M.D. Ala. 1981).

51. *Multicare Medical Center v. State of Washington,* W.D. Wa. C88-421Z (1991); *Pinnacle Nursing Home v. Axelrod,* 719 F. Supp. 1173 (1990); and *Health Care Association of Michigan v. Babcock,* W.D. MI, K89-50063 (1990).

52. *Wilder v. Virginia Hospital Association,* 496 U.S. 498 (1990).

53. Teresa A. Coughlin, Leighton Ku, and John Holahan, *Medicaid since 1980: Costs, Coverage, and the Shifting Alliance between the Federal Government and the States* (Washington, D.C.: Urban Institute Press, 1994), p. 128.

54. Ibid., p. 136.

55. Several actual examples of these techniques are found in General Account-

ing Office, "Medicaid: States Use Illusory Approaches to Shift Costs to Federal Government," *GAO/HEHS-94-133* (August 1994).

56. John Holahan et al., "Explaining the Recent Growth in Medicaid Spending," p. 189.

57. The study was first released as a report for the Kaiser Commission on the Future of Medicaid, entitled *The Medicaid Cost Explosion: Causes and Consequences* (1993). The study was then released in article form in John Holahan, Diane Rowland, Judith Feder, and David Heslam, "Explaining the Recent Growth in Medicaid Spending," *Health Affairs* vol. 12, no. 3 (Fall 1993), pp. 177–193.

58. The remaining 5 percent was due to increased payments to HMOs and increased payments to Medicare for the premiums of persons eligible for both Medicaid and Medicare. John Holahan et al., "Explaining the Recent Growth in Medicaid Spending," p. 182.

59. General Accounting Office, "Medicaid: Spending Pressures Drive States toward Program Reinvention," *GAO/HEHS-95-122* (April 1995), Table 3-1, p. 37.

60. The National Association of Community Health Centers has sued, claiming that federal regulators lack the authority to waive the cost-based reimbursement requirement. *National Association of Community Health Centers v. Shalala* (94 CVO 1238, D.D.C., filed June, 1994).

61. V. O. Key, *Southern Politics in State and Nation* (New York: Random House, 1949).

62. Duane Lockard, *New England State Politics* (Princeton, NJ: Princeton University Press, 1959).

63. John H. Fenton, *Midwest Politics* (New York: Holt, Rinehart and Winston, 1966).

64. Richard E. Dawson and James A. Robinson, "Inter-Party Competition, Economic Variables, and Welfare Policies in the American States," *Journal of Politics* vol. 25 (1963), pp. 265–289.

65. Thomas R. Dye, *Politics, Economics, and the Public: Policy Outcomes in the American States* (Chicago: Rand McNally, 1966).

66. Daniel J. Elazar, *American Federalism: A View from the States* (New York: Thomas Y. Crowell, 1966; 2d edition).

67. Ibid., p. vii.

68. See, for example, Charles Johnson, "Political Culture in American States: Elazar's Formulation Examined," *American Journal of Political Science* vol. 20, no. 3 (August 1976).

69. There were exceptions. In 1969, for example, a few researchers developed models that suggested both politics and economics are important variables. Charles F. Cnudde and Donald McCrone, "Party Competition and Welfare Policies in the American States," *American Political Science Review* vol. 63 (September

1969), pp. 858–866; Ira Sharkansky and Richard I. Hofferbert, "Dimensions of State Politics, Economics and Public Policy," *American Political Science Review,* vol. 63 (September 1969), pp. 867–879.

70. Paul Peterson and Mark Rom, for example, developed a model which demonstrated that "states that are more prosperous, more politically competitive, and culturally more disposed toward redistribution are likely to increase welfare benefits over time and in comparison to other states. But high and increasing poverty levels lead to cuts in welfare. High benefit levels also expose states to welfare-induced migration of the poor." Paul Peterson and Mark Rom, "American Federalism, Welfare Policy and Residential Choices," *American Political Science Review* vol. 83, no. 3 (September 1989), p. 725.

71. Charles J. Barrilleaux and Mark E. Miller, "The Political Economy of State Medicaid Policy," *American Political Science Review* vol. 82 (December 1988), p. 1099.

72. Saundra K. Schneider, "Social Policy-Making in the American States: The Case of AFDC and Medicaid," a paper presented at the 1990 annual meeting of the American Political Science Association, San Francisco, CA, August 30–September 2, 1990.

73. Robert Buchanan, Joseph Cappelleri and Robert Ohsfeldt, "The Social Environment and Medicaid Expenditures: Factors Influencing the Level of State Medicaid Spending," *Public Administration Review* vol. 51, no. 1 (Jan./Feb. 1991) (Medicaid variation is best explained by state income, prior spending levels, and administrative structure); Russell L. Hanson, "Medicaid and the Politics of Redistribution," *American Journal of Political Science* vol. 28, no. 2 (May 1984) (Medicaid variation is best explained by political culture, though interparty competition and medical group influence are factors also); John F. Holahan and Joel W. Cohen, *Medicaid: The Trade-off between Cost-Containment and Access to Care* (Washington, D.C.: The Urban Institute Press, 1986) (Medicaid variation is best explained by state wealth, political culture, number of doctors, and race).

74. Malcolm Goggin, *Policy Design and the Politics of Implementation* (Knoxville: University of Tennessee Press, 1987).

Chapter 4

1. General Accounting Office, "Medicaid: Spending Pressures Drive States toward Program Reinvention," *GAO/HEHS-95-122* (April 1995), Table 1.1, p. 18.

2. Ibid.

3. B. Hyink, S. Brown, and D. Provist, *Politics and Government in California* (New York: Harper and Row, 1989), p. 18.

4. In 1850, for example, women constituted only 8 percent of California's population. *Encyclopaedia Britannica.*

5. John W. Caughy, *California* (New Jersey: Prentice Hall, 1953; 2d edition), pp. 449–450.

6. Other than the civil war pension program (which provided pensions to Union veterans), the federal government had no role in the nation's social welfare system.

7. Herbert Croly, *Progressive Democracy*, pp. 355–356.

8. The courts may ultimately hold that parts of Proposition 166 are unconstitutional. The state legislature, however, cannot itself reverse the voters' commands.

9. Congressional Research Service, *Medicaid Source Book*, Table III-6, p. 194.

10. Ibid., p. 172, Table III-1.

11. Ibid., p. 257.

12. Ibid., p. 172, Table III-1.

13. Ibid., p. 257.

14. David Ellis, *New York State and City* (Ithaca, NY: Cornell University Press, 1979).

15. Ibid., pp. 89–93.

16. Wallace Sayre and Herbert Kaufman, *Governing New York City* (New York: Russell Sage Foundation, 1960).

17. Ellis, *New York State and City*.

18. Robert Stevens and Rosemary Stevens, *Welfare Medicine in America: A Case Study of Medicaid* (New York: The Free Press, 1974), p. 86.

19. Alan Hevesi, *Legislative Politics in New York* (New York: Praeger Press, 1975), p. 120.

20. Ibid., p. 117; Stevens and Stevens, *Welfare Medicine in America*, p. 94.

21. Stevens and Stevens, *Welfare Medicine in America*, p. 163.

22. Ibid., p. 121.

23. Congressional Research Service, *Medicaid Source Book*, Table III-6, pp. 194–195.

24. General Accounting Office, "Medicaid: Spending Pressures Drive States toward Program Reinvention," *GAO/HEHS-95-122* (April 1995), Table 1.1, p. 18.

Chapter 5

1. New York State Majority Task Force on Aging in the 21st Century, *Health Care for a Graying Population: The Coming Crisis?* (Albany, NY: December 1988), p. 56; William Thomas, *Nursing Homes and Public Policy: Drift and Decision in New York State* (Ithaca, N.Y.: Cornell University Press, 1969), p. xiii.

2. New York State Majority Task Force on Aging, *Health Care for a Graying Population*, p. 56.

3. Bruce Vladeck, *Unloving Care: The Nursing Home Tragedy* (New York: Basic Books, 1980), p. 25.

4. Ibid., p. 34.

5. Thomas, *Nursing Homes and Public Policy,* p. 49; Vladeck, *Unloving Care,* p. 36.

6. Thomas, *Nursing Homes and Public Policy,* p. xii.

7. The Urban Institute, *Understanding the Growth in Nursing Home Care, 1964–1974* (Washington, D.C.: Urban Institute, April 1978), Appendix A, p. A-4.

8. Thomas, *Nursing Homes and Public Policy,* p. 98; Vladeck, *Unloving Care,* p. 40.

9. Stevens and Stevens, *Welfare Medicine in America,* p. 23.

10. Thomas, *Nursing Homes and Public Policy,* p. 115; Vladeck, *Unloving Care,* p. 42.

11. Vladeck, *Unloving Care,* p. 46.

12. The 1963 and 1977 figures are from Vladeck, *Unloving Care,* p. 102. The 1993 figure is from Richard DuNah, Jr., Charlene Harrington, Barbara Bedney, and Helen Carrillo, "Variation and Trends in State Nursing Facility Capacity: 1978–93," *Health Care Financing Review* (Fall 1995), p. 188.

13. In 1990, for example, private long-term care insurance policies paid only 1 percent of the nation's nursing home bill. Congressional Research Service, *Medicaid Source Book,* Figure C-3, p. 824.

14. Ibid.

15. In New York City, the average rate is even higher: $142 per day. New York State Department of Health, *Bureau of RHCF Reimbursement: Average 1991 Rates by DOH Region* (Unpublished report, June 12, 1991).

16. Joseph Klun, Rate Development Branch, California Department of Health Services, telephone interview with author June 7, 1991.

17. General Accounting Office, "Nursing Homes: Admission Problems for Medicaid Recipients and Attempts to Solve Them," *GAO/HRD-90-135* (September 1990), p. 30.

18. William McCann, former Assistant Commissioner of the New York State Department of Health and former Director of the New York State Council on Health Care Financing, interview with author, October 16, 1990; The Urban Institute, *Understanding the Growth in Nursing Home Care,* p. F-5.

19. William McCann, interview with author, October 16, 1990.

20. Ibid.

21. Frederick O. R. Hayes, "Nursing Home Care in New York," in *The Impact of National Health Insurance on New York,* ed. M. Lieberman (New York: Prodist, 1977), p. 110.

22. Vladeck, *Unloving Care,* pp. 86–87.

23. State of New York, Office of the State Comptroller, "Staff Study on New York State's Medicaid Program" (March 1989), Schedule G.

24. Ibid., p. 21.

25. Leon Fink and Brian Greenberg, *Upheaval in the Quiet Zone: A History of Hospital Workers Union, Local 1199* (Urbana and Chicago: University of Illinois Press, 1989), p. 113. By 1970, for example, blacks and hispanics made up over 80 percent of hospitals' service and maintenance staffs.

26. Interestingly, however, even in this environment, the effort to organize health care workers was a long and difficult process. This history is summarized nicely in Fink and Greenberg, *Upheaval in the Quiet Zone.*

27. On Lindsay's first day on the job, in 1966, the city's transit workers began a long and disruptive strike.

28. Fink and Greenberg, *Upheaval in the Quiet Zone,* p. 123.

29. Ibid., p. 108.

30. Ibid., pp. 122–128.

31. Vladeck, *Unloving Care,* p. 274.

32. 54 percent were owned by private businessmen, 12 percent by government, and 9 percent by hospitals. Bruce Spitz, *Medicaid Nursing Home Reimbursement: New York, Illinois, and California Case Studies* (Health Care Financing Grants and Contracts Report, October 1981), p. 33.

33. Spitz, *Medicaid Nursing Home Reimbursement,* p. 45.

34. Vladeck, *Unloving Care,* p. 87.

35. Spitz, *Medicaid Nursing Home Reimbursement,* p. 46.

36. At that time, the federal government was responsible for 50 percent of the Medicaid bill, while the state and local counties each contributed 25 percent. In 1982, the state share of long-term care bills was increased to 40 percent, while the county share was reduced to 10 percent.

37. Seymour Budoff, former Director of the New York City Medicaid program, personal communication, July 16, 1990.

38. Many nursing home residents have income marginally above the Medicaid eligibility levels. Such persons can receive Medicaid coverage, however, by paying the nursing home for a portion of their bill. For example, suppose state "A" limits Medicaid coverage to persons with less than $100 in income per month. If Mrs. Smith has income of $150 per month, and a nursing home bill of $1000 per month, Mrs. Smith will pay the home $50 and Medicaid will pay the balance. This process is referred to as "spending down" to Medicaid eligibility.

39. *New York Times* series on nursing home fraud, beginning September 6, 1974.

40. By mid-1975, there were seventeen separate government investigations of the state's nursing home industry.

41. For a good description and discussion of New York City's fiscal crisis, see Robert J. Bailey, *The Crisis Regime* (Albany: State University of New York Press, 1984).

42. Spitz, *Medicaid Nursing Home Reimbursement,* p. 69.

43. Ibid., p. 50.

44. Ibid., p. 57.

45. Fink and Greenberg, *Upheaval in the Quiet Zone*, p. 67.

46. Spitz, *Medicaid Nursing Home Reimbursement*, p. 78.

47. Brian Ellsworth, "An Economic Analysis of the Impact of Government Policies Affecting New York State Nursing Homes" (masters thesis, Cornell University, June 1986), p. 22.

48. Cynthia Rudder, *Case-Mix Reimbursement and the Nursing Home Resident in New York State: Suggestions for Change* (New York: Nursing Home Community Coalition, June 1989).

49. Ellsworth, "An Economic Analysis," p. 21.

50. The New York State Department of Health, *Resource Utilization Groups System* (July 1986), p. 9.

51. New York State Department of Health, "Comparison of 1991 and 1992 RHCF Adjusted Revenue and Expenses" (November 1993), on file with the author.

52. Cynthia Rudder, *Case-Mix Reimbursement and the Nursing Home Resident*.

53. The Urban Institute, *Understanding the Growth in Nursing Home Care*, Appendix A, F-6 and F-27.

54. *California Ass'n of Nursing Homes v. Williams*, 84 Cal. Rept. 590 (Ct. of Appeals, 3d Dist. 1970).

55. Around this same time, California officials were implementing the nation's first Medicaid managed care initiative, described in Chapter 8, under which Medicaid recipients were encouraged to enroll in prepaid health organizations (such as HMOs). California's effort to provide nursing homes with flat-rate reimbursement was also a national trendsetter.

56. Lewin and Associates, "An Evaluation of the Medi-Cal Program's System for Establishing Reimbursement Rates for Nursing Homes" (prepared for the Auditor General of the State of California, October 1987), p. 171.

57. This information includes the District of Columbia.

58. J. Swan, C. Harrington, L. Grant, J. Luehrs and S. Preston, "Trends in Medicaid Nursing Home Reimbursement: 1978–89," *Health Care Financing Review* vol. 14, no. 4 (Summer 1993), p. 126. To be sure, New York's rate covers various services provided only occasionally (such as physical and occupational therapy), while California pays separately for these services. But this variable accounts for only a small amount of the difference in rates.

59. Congressional Research Service, *Medicaid Source Book*, p. 833.

60. State of New York, Office of the State Comptroller, "Staff Study on New York State's Medicaid Program," Schedule G.

61. California Advocates for Nursing Home Reform, *1992 Report Card on California Nursing Homes* (July 1993), p. 6. The disparity between salaries in New

York and those in California is not limited to nurses aides. In 1985, for example, a cook in a New York City nursing home made approximately $10.36 per hour; his counterpart in Los Angeles made approximately $5.17 per hour. State of New York, Office of the State Comptroller, "Staff Study on New York State's Medicaid Program," Schedule G.

62. The Commission on California State Government Organization and Economy (the "Little Hoover Commission"), *The Bureaucracy of Care: Continuing Policy Issues for Nursing Home Services and Regulation* (August 1983).

63. 42 U.S.C. sections 1395i-3(a)–(h) and 42 U.S.C. sections 1396r(a)–(h).

64. 42 U.S.C. section 1396a(a) (13) (A).

65. The two California estimates are cited in a letter from John Rodriguez (deputy director, Department of Health Services) to Gerald Moskowitz (regional administrator, HCFA), dated August 31, 1990, on file with the author. The New York estimate is from personal interviews with Orlando Orozco of the New York State Health Facilities Association, December 5, 1990, and Steven Anderman of the New York State Department of Health, August 16, 1993.

66. *Medi-Cal Long-Term Care Reimbursement Act of 1990* (SB 1087) at 15.

67. Letter from Governor Pete Wilson to President George Bush, February 2, 1991, on file with the author.

68. Letter from Kenneth Kizer (Commissioner, California Department of Health Services) to Gail Wilensky (HCFA Administrator), March 11, 1991, on file with the author.

69. *Valdivia v. Kizer,* Civ. no. S-90-1226 (E.D. Cal., October 11, 1992).

70. *Faulkner and Gray's Medicine and Health* (Washington, D.C.: Faulkner and Gray's Healthcare Information Center, August 9, 1993).

Chapter 6

1. Welfare caseworkers had the discretion to increase a client's cash grant to cover the cost of a range of services. See generally, Title 4A of the *Social Security Act* (the AFDC program) and Title 16 of the *Act* (providing aid to the aged, blind, and disabled). In 1975, funding for such services was consolidated in Title 20 of the *Act*.

2. The Office of National Cost Estimates, U.S. Health Care Financing Administration, "National Health Expenditures: 1988," *Health Care Financing Review* vol. 11, no. 4 (Summer 1990), p. 13.

3. L. Branch, H. Goldberg, V. Cheh, and J. Williams, "Medicare Home Health: A Description of Total Episodes of Care," *Health Care Financing Review* vol. 14, no. 4 (Summer 1993), p. 59.

4. Congressional Research Service, *Medicaid Source Book,* Table II-13, p. 134.

5. Ibid., p. 256, Table V-1.

6. Ibid., pp. 405–406, Table VI-9.

7. Data received from Ann Hallock, New York State Department of Social Services, dated December 28, 1994.

8. Data received from William Schimeck, California Department of Health Services, October 4, 1994.

9. Congressional Research Service, *The Medicaid Source Book,* pp. 41, 44, and 48.

10. Title XX of the *Social Security Act.*

11. Testimony of Loren Suter, California Department of Social Services, August 30, 1990, at the Elder-Care Public Hearing of the Commission of California State Government Organization and Economy.

12. Ann Hallock, New York State Department of Social Services, interview with author, November 28, 1990.

13. Title 3 of the *Revenue Sharing Act of 1972.*

14. New York Social Services Law, section 365-a(2) (c).

15. 18 NYCRR section 505.14(a) (6).

16. New York State Department of Social Services, "Statistical Supplement to the 1989 Annual Report."

17. Barbara Caress, "Home Is Where the Patients Are: New York's Home Care Workers' Contract," *HealthPac Bulletin* vol. 18, no. 3 (Fall 1988), p. 7.

18. Ann Hallock, November 28, 1990, interview.

19. *New York Times,* December 2, 1979.

20. Rebecca Donovan, "Work Stress and Job Satisfaction: A Study of Home Care Workers in New York City," *Home Health Care Services Quarterly* vol. 10 (1989), pp. 100–101.

21. Data received from Ann Hallock, New York State Department of Social Services, dated December 28, 1994.

22. Congressional Research Service, *Medicaid Source Book,* p. 134.

23. S. Crystal, C. Flemming, P. Beck, and G. Smolka, *The Management of Home Care Services* (New York: Springer Publishing Co., 1987), p. 136.

24. The United Hospital Fund, *Home Care in New York City: Providers, Payers, and Clients* (New York: The United Hospital Fund, March 1987), p. 19; Lewin/ ICF, *The Home Care Labor Market in New York State: An Analysis of the Issues and Projection Through 2000* (Washington, D.C.: October 1988), pp. 2–5.

25. Kathryn Haslanger, formerly with the New York City Human Resources Administration, interview with author, April 25, 1990.

26. Crystal et al., *The Management of Home Care Services,* p. 109.

27. Barry Berberich, New York State Department of Social Services, interview with author, June 22, 1991.

28. *The Home Health Services Management and Fiscal Assessment Act of 1991,* New York Social Services Law, 367-j.

29. For example, New York City has yet to implement the fiscal assessment program in its personal care program.

30. Affidavit of Barry Berberich, New York State Department of Social Services, in *Dowd v. Bane,* Index No. 17335-92, dated July 20, 1992, p. 5.

31. United Hospital Fund, "Home Care in New York City," p. 30.

32. New York State Department of Social Services, Statistical Supplement to the 1989 Annual Report.

33. Caress, "Home Is Where the Patients Are," p. 9.

34. Ibid., p. 10.

35. Kathryn Haslanger, formerly with the New York City Human Resources Administration, interview with author, April 25, 1990.

36. Ray Sweeney, New York State Department of Health, interview with author, November 7, 1990.

37. Ibid.

38. Testimony of Loren Suter, California Department of Social Services, August 30, 1991, at the Elder-Care Public Hearings of the Commission on California State Government Organization and Economy.

39. Data received from Ruth Bongiovanni, New York State Department of Social Services, June 24, 1991.

40. State of New York, Office of the State Comptroller, *Staff Study on New York State's Medicaid Program* (March 1989), at Schedule H.

41. Data received from Ann Hallock, New York State Department of Social Services.

42. State of New York, Office of the State Comptroller, *Staff Study on New York State's Medicaid Program* (March 1989), at Schedule H. The other seven states were Ohio, Pennsylvania, Michigan, Illinois, Massachusetts, New Jersey, and Wisconsin.

43. Testimony of Loren Suter, California Department of Social Services, August 30, 1990, at the Elder-Care Public Hearing of the Commission on California State Government Organization and Economy; telephone interview with Fahari Jeffers, of the United Domestic Workers union, September 21, 1994.

44. Data for rural New York and New York City home attendants received from Rosemary Comtompesos, New York State Department of Social Services.

45. Testimony of Loren Suter, California Department of Social Services, August 30, 1990; telephone interview with Fahari Jeffers.

46. Commission on California State Government Organization and Economy (the "Little Hoover Commission"), "Unsafe in Their Own Homes: State Programs Fail to Protect Elderly From Indignity, Abuse and Neglect" (Sacramento, CA: The Little Hoover Commission, November 1991), p. 5.

47. County officials are responsible for the day-to-day administration of the home attendant program. State officials, however, control the amount of state and federal dollars that support program activities and set overall program policy as well.

48. Jerry Rose, Program Manager of California's In-Home Supportive Services Program, interview conducted by Hale Zukos, of the World Institute on Disability, on file with the author.

49. Testimony of Derrell Kelch, California Association of Homes for the Aging, August 30, 1990, at the Elder-Care Public Hearing of the Commission on California State Government Organization and Economy.

50. Shelly Rouillard, formerly with the California Rural Legal Assistance Foundation, interview with author, September 6, 1990.

51. A 1987 report issued by the California Auditor General estimated that approximately 7 percent of all IHSS workers had prior criminal records. This report was cited during the testimony of Nathan Shapell, Chairman, Commission on California State Government Organization and Economy, during the Elder-Care Public Hearing, held on August 30, 1990.

52. Charlene Harrington and Leslie A. Grant, "The Delivery, Regulation, and Politics of Home Care: A California Case Study," *The Gerontologist* vol. 30, no. 4 (1990), at Table 1.

53. Crystal et al., *The Management of Home Care Services,* p. 4; and David L. Rabin and Patricia Stockton, *Long-Term Care for the Elderly: A Factbook* (Oxford: Oxford University Press, 1987), p. 140.

54. Commission of California State Government Organization and Economy, "Unsafe in Their Own Homes," p. 4.

55. Lewin/ICF, "The Home Care Labor Market in New York State," pp. 2–5.

56. 42 C.F.R. section 440.170(f) (3).

57. Clients could claim in an administrative review process that the cutback would impose irreparable harm. But the burden of proof is on the client.

58. The number of home health agencies in the state is set forth in C. Harrington, L. Grant, S. Ingman, and S. Mildner, "The Study of Regulation of Home Health Care Agencies in Two States: California and Missouri" (Working Paper, Institute for Health and Aging: University of California at San Francisco, December 1988), p. 9. The number of agencies participating routinely in Medi-Cal is set forth in R. Brown and G. Dallek, "Changing Health Care in Los Angeles: Poverty amid Affluence, Competition Leading to Crisis" (March 1990), p. 72.

59. Testimony of Joseph Hafkenschiel, California Association for Health Services at Home, August 12, 1987, before the Assembly Committee on Aging and Long-Term Care.

60. The various state figures are reported in State of New York, Office of the State Comptroller, at Schedule H.

Chapter 7

1. Paul Starr, *The Transformation of American Medicine* (New York: Basic Books, 1982), p. 155.

2. Ibid., p. 74.

3. G. Annas, S. Law, R. Rosenblatt, and K. Wing, *American Health Law* (Boston: Little, Brown and Co., 1990), p. 10.

4. *The Hospital Survey and Construction Act of 1946* (generally referred to as the *Hill-Burton Act*).

5. Eli Ginzberg, *From Health Dollars to Health Services* (New Jersey: Rowman and Allanheld, 1986), pp. 130–131.

6. C. Brecher, K. Thorpe, and C. Green, "New York City Health and Hospitals Corporation," in *Competition and Compassion: Conflicting Roles for Public Hospitals,* ed. S. Altman, C. Brecher, M. Henderson, and K. Thorpe (Ann Arbor: Health Administration Press, 1989), p. 46.

7. New York State Council on Health Care Financing, *Recommendations for Financing Hospital Inpatient Care* (October 1980), pp. 38–39.

8. See generally, New York Public Health Law, section 2800 *et seq.*

9. Stevens and Stevens, *Welfare Medicine in America,* p. 110.

10. Even the shortened freeze was subsequently struck down by the courts.

11. New York Public Health Law, section 2807(3).

12. For a discussion of the legislative compromise, see Sylvia A. Law, *Blue Cross: What Went Wrong* (New Haven: Yale University Press, 1974), p. 212 (fn. 572); and The Council on Health Care Financing, *Recommendations for Financing Hospital Inpatient Care,* p. 43 (fn. 14).

13. 10 NYCRR 86.14(b).

14. Law, *Blue Cross,* p. 105.

15. The two dominant unions are Local 1199 of the Retail Workers Union (which organizes in private, nonprofit facilities) and District Council 37 of AFSCME (which organizes in the public hospitals).

16. See Chapter 5 for a longer discussion of Lindsay's and Rockefeller's motives.

17. Leon Fink and Brian Greenberg, *Upheaval in the Quiet Zone: A History of Hospital Workers Union, Local 1199* (Urbana and Chicago: University of Illinois Press, 1989), pp. 122–128.

18. State of New York, Office of the State Comptroller, *Staff Study on New York State's Medicaid Program* (March 1989), p. 11.

19. James R. Knickman and Ann-Marie Foltz, "A Statistical Analysis of Reasons for East-West Differences in Hospital Use," *Inquiry* vol. 22 (Spring 1985), p. 45.

20. Milton I. Roemer and Max Shain, *Hospital Utilization Under Insurance* (Ithaca, N.Y.: Cornell School of Business and Public Administration, 1959), pp. 17–18 and 51, cited in Paul Starr, *The Social Transformation of American Medicine,* p. 487, note 69.

21. Ralph E. Berry Jr., "Prospective Rate Reimbursement and Cost Containment: Formula Reimbursement in New York," *Inquiry* vol. 13, page 3 (Sept. 1976).

22. Kenneth Thorpe, "Health Care," in *The Two New Yorks,* eds. Gerald Benjamin and Charles Brecher (New York: Russell Sage Foundation, 1988), p. 366.

23. Ibid., p. 366.

24. Fink and Greenberg, *Upheaval in the Quiet Zone,* p. 177.

25. William McCann, former Director of the New York State Council on Health Care Financing, interview with author, October 16, 1990.

26. Report of the New York State Council on Health Care Financing (March 31, 1986), p. 20.

27. Kenneth Thorpe, "The American States and Canada: A Comparative Analysis of Health Care Spending," *Journal of Health Politics, Policy and Law* vol. 18, no. 2 (Summer 1993), pp. 477–489.

28. Medicare's new payment system provided teaching facilities with a "direct medical education adjustment" to reimburse hospitals for a portion of residents' and faculty's salaries and with an "indirect medical education adjustment" to reimburse hospitals for the sicker patients and the more rigorous care that is generally associated with teaching facilities. Indeed, Congress was so anxious to protect the teaching facilities that it doubled the indirect adjustment proposed by the federal bureaucrats supervising the program. Louise B. Russell, *Medicare's New Hospital Payment System: Is It Working?* (Washington, D.C.: Brookings Institution, 1989), p. 12.

29. Stuart H. Altman and Christine M. Garfink, *The Impact of the Federal Prospective Payment System on New York's Hospitals* (Waltham, Mass.: Bigel Institute for Health Policy, 1990), p. 6.

30. Materials received from the Hospital Association of New York State, on file with the author.

31. Materials received from the Health Department, on file with the author.

32. *New York Times,* August 1, 1990, p. B-2.

33. California Department of Health Services, *The Medi-Cal Program: A Brief Summary of Major Events* (March 1990).

34. The Aging Health Policy Center, *State Discretionary Policies and Services in the Medicaid, Social Services, and Supplemental Security Income Programs* (University of California at San Francisco, 1983), p. 85.

35. Ibid., p. 171.

36. Sacramento Bee, March 3, 1971, cited in Barry Ensminger, "Beware the Medicaid Cap," *HealthPac Bulletin* vol. 12, no. 8 (November 1981), p. 8.

37. Barry Ensminger, "Beware the Medicaid Cap," p. 7.

38. Ibid., pp. 8–9.

39. See generally, Martha Solish, "Los Angeles County Public Hospitals," in *Competition and Compassion: Conflicting Roles for Public Hospitals,* ed. S. Altman, C. Brecher, M. Henderson, and K. Thorpe (Ann Arbor: Health Administration Press, 1989), p. 97.

40. Linda Bergthold, "Crabs in a Bucket: The Politics of Health Care Reform in California," *The Journal of Health Politics, Policy and Law* vol. 9, no. 2 (Summer 1984), p. 204.

41. *California Hospital Association v. Obledo*, 602 F. 2d 1357 (9th Cir. 1979).

42. *California Hospital Association v. Schweiker*, 559 F. Supp. 110, 117 (C.D. Cal. 1982), *aff'd* 705 F. 2d 466 (9th Cir. 1982).

43. Linda Bergthold, "Crabs in a Bucket," p. 205.

44. In 1990, for example, the occupancy rate in California's hospitals was 64.2 percent; in New York, in contrast, the rate was 86.8 percent. Materials received from the New York State Department of Health, on file with the author.

45. The Aging Health Policy Center, *State Discretionary Policies and Services in the Medicaid, Social Services, and Supplemental Security Income Programs* (University of California at San Francisco, 1983), p. 268.

46. Abt Associates, *Medicaid Program Evaluation: Inpatient Hospital Reimbursement* (Cambridge, Mass.: Abt Associates, 1987).

47. L. Johns, R. Derzon and M. Anderson, *Selective Contracting for Health Services in California: Final Report* (Washington, D.C.: Lewin and Associates and the National Governors' Association, 1985).

48. California Medical Assistance Commission, *Annual Report to the Legislature: January 1993*, pp. 9–11.

49. L. Johns, R. Derzon and M. Anderson, *Selective Contracting for Health Services in California*, p. 41.

50. California Department of Health Services, *Expanding Medi-Cal Managed Care* (Sacramento, CA: California Department of Health Services, 1993), p. 27.

51. Health Care Financing Administration: Division of Medicaid Statistics, "Medicaid State Tables for Fiscal Year 1989," Tables 3 and 11, on file with author.

52. Katharine R. Levit, Helen C. Lazenby, Cathy Cowan, Darleen K. Won, Jean M. Stiller, Lekha Sivarajan, and Madie W. Stewart, "State Health Expenditure Accounts: Building Blocks for State Health Spending Analysis," *Health Care Financing Review* (Fall 1995), p. 250.

53. Prospective Payment Assessment Commission, *Medicare and the American Health Care System — Report to Congress* (June 1995), Table 5-14, p. 133.

54. C. Winterbottom, D. Liska, and K. Obermaier, *State-Level Databook on Health Care Access and Financing* (Washington, D.C.: Urban Institute, 1995), Table F1, p. 156.

55. Ibid., Table F2, p. 157.

Chapter 8

1. Jonathan P. Weiner and Gregory de Lissovoy, "Razing a Tower of Babel: A Taxonomy for Managed Care and Health Insurance Plans," *Journal of Health Politics, Policy and Law* vol. 18 (Spring 1993), p. 77.

2. For a description of the multitude of institutional arrangements that today go under the rubric of "managed care" see note 18 to Chapter Two.

3. Forty-four states have adopted Medicaid managed care initiatives.

4. The Kaiser Commission on the Future of Medicaid, *Medicaid and Managed Care: Lessons from the Literature* (Washington, D.C.: Kaiser Commission on the Future of Medicaid, 1995).

5. The medical safety net includes those hospitals (both public and nonprofit) and community health centers that have traditionally cared for both Medicaid clients and the uninsured, along with a few individual practitioners who serve a primarily indigent population.

6. In 1993, over 50 percent of California's privately insured population was enrolled in HMOs. Prospective Payment Assessment Commission, *Medicare and the American Health Care System: Report to Congress* (June 1995), Table 5-16, p. 136.

7. In 1972, for example, the legislature enacted the *Waxman-Duffy Prepaid Health Plan Act,* which regulated for the first time the marketing activities of the new managed care organizations. Then, in 1975, the legislature enacted the *Knox-Keene Health Care Service Plan Act,* which required the state's Department of Corporations to license all prepaid health plans, including those with Medi-Cal contracts.

8. See, for example, General Accounting Office, *Better Controls Needed for Health Maintenance Organizations under Medicaid in California,* Report # B-164031(3), September 1974; General Accounting Office, *Deficiencies in Determining Payments to Prepaid Health Plans Under California's Medicaid Program,* Report # MWD-76-15, August 1975; and General Accounting Office, *Relationships between Nonprofit Prepaid Health Plans with California Medicaid Contracts and For-Profit Entities Affiliated With Them,* Report # HRD-77-4, November 1976.

9. The law did exempt federally funded community health centers from the 50 percent requirement.

10. Under selective contracting, state officials estimate the number of hospital beds needed for Medi-Cal patients, hospitals bid for Medi-Cal contracts, and hospitals without contracts provide only emergency room care to Medi-Cal patients.

11. Prior to 1985, County Organized Health Systems were exempt from the requirement that no more than 75 percent of an HMOs clients could be on Medicaid and Medicare. Today, the COHSs still in existence (in Santa Barbara, San Mateo, and Solano) have Congressional exemptions from the 75 percent rule.

12. Congressional Research Service, *Medicaid Source Book,* p. 1028.

13. Legal services lawyers representing Medi-Cal clients argued that DHS needed federal permission to implement a default program. While the state disagreed, they ultimately sought federal approval. In November 1993, the federal government okayed the default but urged the state to work with both federal officials and consumer advocates in developing the health care options materials that would be presented to clients at the time of enrollment. As of this writing (August 1994), the default has yet to be implemented, and the health care options materials developed by the state are being challenged in federal court.

14. Federal legislation enacted in 1981 required states to "take into account" the situation of those hospitals that serve a disproportionate number of low-income persons. Despite this command, however, many states refused to provide the subsidies. In 1987, Congress required states to provide subsidies to hospitals that met federally defined criteria. The 1987 law went into effect in 1990.

15. Of the key interest groups it might be helpful to note the most influential organizations. Of the hospital organizations, they are the California Association of Health and Hospital Systems and the California Association of Public Hospitals. The most influential HMO organization is the California Association of HMOs. Interestingly, Foundation is the state's only large HMO that doesn't belong to the Association. The most influential group of doctors is the California Medical Association. The most influential group of community clinics is the California Health Foundation. And, finally, the most influential advocates are the Western Center on Law and Poverty, the National Health Law Project, and the Service Employees and Industrial Union.

16. The basis for the hundred thousand figure was a series of telephone calls, made by Jonathan Lewis, then the Executive Director of CAHMO, in which numerous HMOs agreed to enroll small numbers of additional Medi-Cal clients. At that time, the industry was quite reluctant to accept Medi-Cal clients, and the hundred thousand figure was considered high. Soon thereafter, however, as health care reformers emphasized managed competition and managed care, the HMOs willingness to accept Medi-Cal clients increased, and CAHMO officials declared the hundred thousand figure to be a floor, not a cap.

17. Federal officials have since used this audit to demand the return of $5 million dollars. This federal claim remains unresolved.

18. The California Medical Assistance Commission conducted these negotiations.

19. The six, one of whom worked for DHS's parent agency, the California Health and Welfare Agency, were of course in regular contact with their bureaucratic supervisors.

20. There were originally supposed to be thirteen county participants, but San Diego County was later authorized to implement a program, modeled after geographic managed care, in which several HMOs compete for the Medi-Cal business.

21. Personal interviews with Jonathan Lewis, director of the L.A. Health Advantage, and former director of the California Association of HMOs, February 9, 1994; Bill Caswell, of Maxi-Care, February 14, 1994; and Michael Owens, of Cigna, February 14, 1994.

22. Health Care Financing Administration, "Request for Additional Information on the Two-Plan Model" (San Francisco, CA: Sept. 1995), on file with author.

23. Health Care Financing Administration, "Report on Medi-Cal Managed Care" (San Francisco, CA: 1994), on file with author.

24. General Accounting Office, "Medicaid Managed Care: More Competition and Oversight Would Improve California's Expansion Plan," *GAO/HEHS-95-87* (April 1995).

25. Article 28 of New York's Public Health Law prohibits investor-owned hospitals from operating in New York. Prior to 1985, this law was interpreted to also prohibit investor-owned HMOs.

26. John Holahan, Martcia Wade, Michael Gates, and Lynn Tsoflias, "The Impact of Medicaid Adoption of the Medicare Fee Schedule," *Health Care Financing Review* vol. 14 (Spring 1993), p. 15.

27. Eli Ginzberg, "Improving Health Care for the Poor: Lessons from the 1980s," *Journal of the American Medical Association* vol. 271, no. 6 (February 9, 1994), p. 465.

28. James Swan, Charlene Harrington, Leslie Grant, John Luehrs, and Steve Preston, "Trends in Medicaid Nursing Home Reimbursement: 1978–89," *Health Care Financing Review* vol. 14 (Summer 1993), p. 126.

29. Prospective Payment Assessment Commission, *Medicaid Hospital Payment Congressional Report: C-91-02* (October 1, 1991), p. 33.

30. While Medi-Cap ended, around eight thousand Medicaid clients chose to remain with their managed care provider on a voluntary basis.

31. Sarah Liebschutz, *Bargaining Under Federalism* (Albany, N.Y.: SUNY Press, 1991), p. 169.

32. Research Triangle Institute, Center for Health Research, *Nationwide Evaluation of Medicaid Competition Demonstrations, Volume 7,* "Analysis of Administrative Costs in the Medicaid Competition Demonstrations," HCFA Contract 50-83-500 (May 31, 1988), p. 70; New York State Department of Social Services and the Center for Development of Human Services (at Buffalo State College), "Process Review of the Monroe County Medi-Cap Program" (undated document on file with the author), p. 5.

33. The BHP is exempt from the federal requirement that 25 percent of an HMO's clients not be on Medicaid or Medicare.

34. The New York figures are from Paul Tenan of the New York State Department of Health, in an interview with author on July 13, 1993, and Katherine Allen of the New York State HMO Conference, in an interview with author on July 19, 1993. The California figures are from Bill Caswell of MaxiCare, in an interview with author on February 14, 1994, and Michael Owens of Cigna, in an interview with author also on February 14, 1994.

35. Ironically, state officials enacted the law as a way of raising an estimated $35 million in revenue; the impact on HMO behavior was (by most accounts) an unintended benefit.

36. The surcharge was struck down both by a federal district court in New York and by the 2d circuit court of appeals. In May 1995, however, the Supreme Court

reversed the lower court decisions and held that the surcharge did not violate ERISA. *New York State Conference on Blue Cross and Blue Shield Plans v. Travelers Ins. Co.,* 115 S. Ct. 1671 (1995).

37. Elisabeth Rosenthal, "Albany to Require Improvements in Service by Medicaid HMOs," *New York Times,* November 17, 1995, p. A-1.

38. Ian Fisher and Esther Fein, "Forced Marriage of Medicaid and Managed Care Hits Snags," *New York Times,* August 28, 1995, p. B-1.

39. To be sure, not all of the key players are well established. In New York, for example, Managed Health Care Systems has evolved primarily to participate in this competition.

40. Adverse selection occurs when HMOs enroll low-risk low-cost clients, leaving the high-cost clients for others. HMOs (and other insurers) often market their product only to their preferred customers. The best way to eliminate adverse selection would be to implement an effective system of risk adjustment (paying HMOs with high-risk clients more than those with low-risk clients). But since the technology of risk adjustment is still in its infancy, states need to regulate closely HMO marketing and enrollment patterns.

Chapter 9

1. See especially James Madison, *The Federalist,* No. 10, written soon after the Constitutional Convention.

2. Andrew Dobelstein, *Politics, Economics and the Public Welfare* (Englewood, N.J.: Prentice Hall, 1986), p. 2.

3. Jill Quadagno, "From Old-Age Assistance to Supplemental Security Income: The Political Economy of Relief in the South, 1935–1972," in *The Politics of Social Policy in the United States,* ed. M. Weir, A. Orloff, and T. Skocpol (Princeton, N.J.: Princeton University Press, 1988).

4. Richard P. Nathan, "Federalism: The Great Composition," in *The New American Political System, 2d Edition,* ed. Anthony King (Washington, D.C., American Enterprise Institute 1990), pp. 231–261.

5. Eric Nordlinger, *On The Autonomy of the Democratic State* (Cambridge, MA: Harvard University Press, 1981).

6. Gabriel A. Almond, "The Return to the State," *American Political Science Review* vol. 82, no. 3 (September 1988).

7. James A. Morone, "The Bureaucracy Empowered," in *The Politics of Health Care Reform: Lessons from the Past, Prospects for the Future,* eds. James A. Morone and Gary S. Belkin (Durham and London: Duke University Press, 1994), pp. 148–164.

8. Ibid. at 148.

9. Lawrence D. Brown, "Adventures in Governance: Policy Culture and Health Reform Politics," a paper prepared for a Woodrow Wilson School Conference, held at Princeton University, November 1995.

10. Ibid.

11. Thomas R. Oliver, "Analysis, Advice, and Congressional Leadership: The Physician Payment Review Commission and the Politics of Medicare," *Journal of Health Politics, Policy and Law* vol. 18, no. 1 (Spring 1993), pp. 113–174.

12. Mark A. Peterson, "Congress in the 1990s: From Iron Triangles to Policy Networks," in *The Politics of Health Care Reform: Lessons from the Past, Prospects for the Future,* eds. James A. Morone and Gary S. Belkin (Durham and London: Duke University Press, 1994), pp. 103–147.

13. Robert B. Hackey, "Regulatory Regimes and State Health Policy," in *The Politics of Health Care Reform: Lessons from the Past, Prospects for the Future,* eds. James A. Morone and Gary S. Belkin (Durham and London: Duke University Press, 1994), pp. 418–429.

14. Malcolm Goggin, *Policy Design and the Politics of Implementation* (Knoxville: University of Tennessee Press, 1987).

15. Frank J. Thompson, "Critical Challenges to State and Local Public Service," in *Revitalizing State and Local Public Service: Strengthening Performance, Accountability, and Citizen Confidence,* ed. Frank J. Thompson (San Francisco: Jossey-Bass 1993), p. 11.

16. Deborah Stone, "State Innovation in Health Policy," a paper prepared for the Ford Foundation Conference on "The Fundamental Questions of Innovation," held at Duke University (May 1991), p. 26.

17. A good starting point for a new intergovernmental health care compact is set forth in The Second Report of the National Commission on the State and Local Public Service, *Frustrated Federalism–Rx for State and Local Health Care Reform* (Albany, N.Y.: Rockefeller Institute of Government, 1993), pp. 57–65.

18. Congressional Budget Office, *Universal Health Insurance Coverage Using Medicare's Payment Rates* (Washington, D.C.: U.S. Government Printing Office, 1991).

19. Jerry Mashaw proposes this model for the United States. Jerry L. Mashaw, "Taking Federalism Seriously: The Case for State-Led Health Care Reform," *Domestic Affairs* vol. 2 (1993/94), p. 12.

Index

Introduction

Having cholesterol levels that are higher than normal puts you at risk for cardiovascular disease. High cholesterol levels in the blood will eventually lead to clogged arteries that can cause a blockage to the heart or to the brain. If these arteries become clogged, it can produce a stroke or a heart attack. If a person is diagnosed with high cholesterol and does not change their diet the high cholesterol will have detrimental effects on their health. If you do nothing about your cholesterol and it is highly possible a stroke or heart attack will happen in the future. Dieting is one of the best ways to correct high cholesterol and both the low carb and the Paleolithic diet plans are excellent to help lower the cholesterol naturally.

Many physicians and health care providers agree that the first line of action when the blood cholesterol levels are elevated is to change the diet. Dieting alone can often lower the cholesterol levels back to normal. Low carb foods, which are found in the low carb diet and the Paleolithic diet, are the right foods to eat to help the body to bring the cholesterol levels back to normal. Both of the diets feature foods that are lean meats (high proteins) and fresh fruits and vegetables, in particular green leafy vegetables. If you are accustomed to a diet of high carbs it means you probably have an addiction to junk food. Junk foods are high in carbs and contain a lot of sugar and empty calories. A junk food diet will help to raise cholesterol levels.

The body needs fiber to help cleanse the body and lower the cholesterol. Both the low carb diet and the Paleolithic diet have the fiber from fruits and vegetables. Fiber from vegetables is one of the best ways the body can receive this necessary nutrient.

Most of the foods included in the low carb diet plan and the Paleolithic diet plan are considered "super foods." These are foods that highly nutritious and help the body to function better, including maintaining a better cholesterol level. "Good" fats, which make up a large portion of the low carb diet plan, help the body to have a stronger immune system and be better able to fight off the illnesses caused by high cholesterol.

If you have been diagnosed with high cholesterol and your health care provider encouraged you to try dieting and changing your diet to lower the cholesterol levels you may want to show them this book. Let them see the recipes included in the low carb diet plan and the Paleolithic diet plan and ask them if the foods included in the book are ones that will help your body to lower your cholesterol levels naturally. Chances are they will say yes and give you their seal of approval on both of diets as good diets to help lower your cholesterol.

It is wise when dieting to lower cholesterol to make the diet a permanent lifestyle change. You will find so many recipes within this book between the low carb diet plan and the Paleolithic diet plan that you can plan the meals for weeks without repeating the dishes. There are even healthy snack and dessert recipes.

When going on a diet to help improve a health condition it is important to stick with the diet plan and not cheat. With all the wonderful recipes in this book, there is no reason to cheat. You can find recipes that probably include all your favorite (healthy) foods. If you have a strong addiction to junk food, you need to break that bad habit. By feeding your body nutritious foods from the low carb diet plan and the Paleolithic diet plan, you are helping your body to break the junk food habit. Before too much longer you will no longer crave the junk and instead you will want to eat the healthy foods.

Ironically, skipping meals is not a good idea if you are

attempting to become healthier. Your body needs food for the energy to be able to function. When cholesterol levels are high, the body needs the right foods to help bring the cholesterol levels back down to a normal reading. Eat breakfast, lunch, and supper and include snacks in between the meals. Eat small to moderate sized meals, avoid over stuffing. Avoid eating out of habit and only eat when the body feels hungry.

By choosing recipes from this book, from the low carb and the Paleolithic diet plans, you are giving your body the best foods it needs to help heal and strengthen the immune system, which will in turn help the body to regulate the cholesterol levels. You can do more research and find out how "low carb diets help to reduce cholesterol levels." Remember both of the sections in this book are low carb so you are giving your body the best chance to be healthy.

Stick with the diet plan to help lower the cholesterol levels. The food you eat may be responsible for your elevated cholesterol levels. Smoking will also raise the cholesterol levels. Genetics also plays a role in some people for elevated levels. No matter where you fall, if your cholesterol is on the rise you must stop your bad habits, quit smoking, and eat better. It is much better for the body if dieting alone can lower the levels. If not, there are prescription medications, but they do come with risks. Do all you can before going on medications to lower your cholesterol naturally.

Always clear your diet plan with your health care provider. The low carb diet and the Paleolithic diet both show promise to help start and maintain a healthy eating lifestyle. Both of the diets have helped others to lower their cholesterol naturally if they stuck with the diet plan. Take your health care provider's advice with your health, especially if they suggested a change in your diet. When you receive a high cholesterol reading, normally you can diet for a couple of months to help bring it down. Keep the diet changes you make and keep your cholesterol levels normal.

Section 1: Low Carb Diet

Low calorie diet is a general phrase that can have different meanings. Anyone can eat smaller portions of the same foods they are already consuming, but this doesn't adequately justify a low calorie diet. What you eat makes a huge difference in getting the most out of any type of diet. Advertising trends can misrepresent the true meaning of a low calorie diet, while staying within certain truthful perimeters. This book is designed to bring focus on true low calorie diets, that introduce you to a new way of life. Being stronger, healthier and having more energy, is the goal of a successful low calorie diet.

There will be misconceptions addressed, as you read through the chapters. Facts about preservatives, sugar, grains and drinks, will awaken your thoughts about what you are feeding yourself, and your family. The truth is, a low calorie diet is not just for losing weight, but learning how all foods have a direct effect on your body. Just as you know that cigarettes and large amounts of alcohol are harmful, habits of eating certain foods can weaken you immune system, slow down metabolism, and cause fatty tissue to form in your arteries and veins.

You will also find delicious recipes that are just right for stepping into your new life. If you wish to shed a few pounds, mix and match the recipes and portions, according to the carbs. With each recipe made from low-carb foods, and under 500 calories each, the choices are huge.

Why Calorie Counting is a Lie

Keeping calories low should not involve taking out a book and writing down every calorie of food you eat. That gets real boring, real fast. You simply need to know what types of foods can easily be burned off and which ones, cannot. One of the highest forms of calories that is difficult to unload, is sugar. Look at any label and you will see this word.

According to the American Heart Association, no more than 100 calories of sugar should make up a grown woman's diet in one day. This amounts to 6 teaspoons. For a man, 150 calories, or 9 teaspoons, should be the limit. One bowl of whole-grain cereal with milk, contains as much as 9 teaspoons of sugar.

While this may seem downhearted, it gets even worse. Preservatives play a very important role in adding empty calories and high carbs. Take, for example, a box of macaroni and cheese. You may feel that you are being frugal in selecting a product that has cheese, grain, and vitamins, not to mention a shelf life of a year, but here is the ugly truth. Preservatives contain corn syrup, hydrogenated oil, nitrates or sulfates. While consumption of these ingredients can give you a sensation of fullness, they are very difficult for the digestive system to process. Feeling sluggish, developing heart burn and producing fat, are three real symptoms of consuming processed foods. While the package calories may read, 400 calories per serving, is doesn't tell you that these calories are close to impossible to burn off.

You can make it a habit of counting calories, but unless you start with foods that are good for your body, consuming a low carb diet, will be in vein.

Chapter 1: Rise and Shine with a Fortified Breakfast

Crunchy Maple Grape Nuts

Description

Breakfast should contain energy-packed foods to jump start your day. However, in the hustle and bustle of preparing for the day, many people grab a box of cereal. Instead of breaking this habit, keep your own homemade varieties on hand. Low calorie and delicious, these recipes will give your family the right mix of vitamins in a low carb diet. Make ahead and store in airtight containers.

Yields: 12 Servings

Ingredients

3 cups whole wheat flour
1/2 cup barley flour
1/3 cup oat flour
1/3 cup toasted wheat germ
1/2 cup brown sugar

1/2 teaspoon salt

2 teaspoons baking soda

2 teaspoons maple flavoring

1/4 cup heated honey or maple syrup

1/2 cup low-fat milk

2 teaspoons cinnamon

Instructions

1. Warm oven to 325 degrees.

2. Sift and blend dry ingredients

3. In a separate bowl, beat the liquid ingredients together.

4. Stir liquid ingredients into dry ingredients.

5. If the mixture is too watery, work in additional flour.

6, Spread on 2 or 3 baking sheets and bake for 10-15 minutes. After baking, allow to cool, then break up any large clumps and return to oven for an additional 10 minutes.

7. Cool and store in air-tight container.

Healthy Honey Oat Cereal

Description

Here is another version of homemade cereal for those that love to wake up their mouths with lots of crunch and flavor. Nuts, raisins and sweet natural ingredients make this breakfast cereal a great kick start to the day.

Yields: 12 Servings

Ingredients

4 1/2 cups rolled oats
6 Tablespoons sunflower seeds
12 Tablespoons sliced almonds
6 Tablespoons chopped pecans
6 Tablespoons raisins
6 Tablespoons honey
1/4 teaspoon cinnamon
1/4 teaspoon maple extract

Instructions

1. Warm oven to 325 degrees.

2. Place a small pan over a larger pan of boiling water

and add the honey, cinnamon and extract. Heat just until well mixed.

3. Spread baking sheet with aluminum foil and combine all other ingredients (except raisins). You may want to use a baking pan that has a slight lip around the sides, or raise up the edges of the foil to keep dry ingredients from falling off.

4. Using your hands, or a large wooden spoon, mix well, the dry ingredients.

5. Add the honey mixture and coat as much of the dry ingredients as you can.

6. Spread the mixture evenly over the pan and bake for 15 minutes.

7. Remove from oven and let cool. Do not worry if your cereal does not appear crunchy. This comes once it has cooled.

9. After cooling, mix in the raisins and store in an airtight container.

French Toast Strawberry Dippers

Description

Getting kids to the breakfast table is a tough chore. Usually running late, they will grab a finger food, like a doughnut or other gluten-filled treat. Have these quick dippers ready to reach for as they hit the door, and know that they are getting good taste and healthy energy.

Yields: 4 Servings

Ingredients

- 8 slices low-carb sandwich white bread
- 4 Tablespoons softened cream cheese
- 6 fresh, sliced strawberries
- 3 large eggs
- 1/4 cup low-fat milk
- 1 Tablespoon butter
- 1/2 cup maple syrup
- 1/4 cup no-sugar strawberry jam

Instructions

1. Spread cream cheese on 4 slices of bread.

2. Line the cream cheese topping with the sliced strawberries.

3. Top with a bread slice to make a sandwich.

4. In a bowl, mix together the eggs and milk.

5. Use 1/2 of the butter to lightly grease a griddle or skillet and heat on medium.

6. Dip the sandwiches into the egg batter, one at a time, and place in the warmed griddle or skillet.

7. Cook the bread on each side until golden brown. Add remaining butter, if needed.

8. Remove each sandwich, pat with paper towels and cut into 4 long sections.

9. Combine the syrup and jam and heat in a microwave for 30 seconds.

10. Remove and stir well.

11. Place the tasty toast sections in a bread basket, beside the dip, and watch them disappear.

Breakfast Egg Muffins

Description

Use the weekend to cook up a filling and healthy egg breakfast for the day ahead. It will soon become a tradition of a starting a free day, just right, with plenty to go around.

Yields: 8 Servings

Ingredients

8 eggs
½ cup Swiss or Cheddar cheese
½ cup milk
¼ cup chopped onion
¼ cup chopped mushrooms
¼ cup green pepper
¼ cup chopped tomatoes
2 Tablespoons butter
4 plain bagels
8 stale pieces of bread

Instructions

1. Lay out the pieces of bread and cut out the middle in

the shape of a circle. This will serve as a pattern for cooking your egg mixture.

2. In a bowl, whisk the eggs and milk together.

3. Blend in the onion, mushrooms, green pepper and tomatoes.

4. Melt 1 Tablespoon butter in a large skillet and arrange the bread patterns.

5. Pour the egg mixture in the center of each bread pattern, lower heat and cover.

6. After about 4 minutes, remove the cover and sprinkle each round egg with cheese.

7. Add extra butter if needed to keep the bottoms from sticking.

7. Turn off heat and recover skillet.

8. Toast ½ bagel and place on a plate.

9. Carefully remove each egg and peel away the outer bread.

10. Place the round egg on top of the bagel, discarding the bread.

Serve with fresh fruit or a glass of juice.

Cinnamon Raisin Muffins

Description

Nothing can compare to fresh, homemade muffins, right from the oven. These treats will satisfy your craving for bread and sweets, but actually give you less than 150 calories each. Vary the ingredients and have a different selection of muffins each week.

Yields: 12 Servings

Ingredients

1 ½ cups flour
1 ½ teaspoons baking powder
½ teaspoon baking soda
¼ cup butter, refrigerated
1 egg
¼ cup sour cream
¼ cup milk
¼ cup raisins
2 Tablespoons sugar, or sugar substitute
1 teaspoon cinnamon

Instructions

1. Heat oven to 400 degrees F.

2. Combine flour, baking powder and baking soda in large bowl.

3. Cut in the butter until coarse crumbs form.

4. Make a well in the center.

5. In a small bowl, beat the egg, then add the sour cream, milk, raisins, sugar and cinnamon, blending thoroughly.

6. Pour the egg mixture in the center of the flour and mix well.

7. Take a muffin pan and either line with paper muffin holders, or grease lightly.

8. Fill each cup 2/3 full.

9. Bake for 15 minutes, or until browned.

Apple butter or fruit preserves can be used to spread on each muffin.

Asparagus and Mushroom Omelet

Description

This dish makes a meaty and tasty meal for not only breakfast, but lunch, as well. With only 5 grams of carbohydrates and 21 grams of protein, per serving, you will pick up extra energy and not get hungry through the course of the day.

Yields: 4 Servings

Ingredients

8 eggs
8 Tablespoons water
12 stalks fresh asparagus
1 cup sliced mushrooms
1 cup low-fat mozzarella cheese

Instructions

1. In a large skillet, add an inch of water and bring to a boil.

2. Add the asparagus, in two or three different sections, and cook uncovered, just until tender-crisp. Remove and

pat dry.

3. Using a large bowl, whisk the eggs and water.

4. Prepare a large skillet by melting 1 Tablespoon butter

.

5. When butter reaches a sizzle over medium-high heat, add ½ of the egg mixture.

6. Cook until the bottom of the egg mixture sets.

7. Carefully lift up the edges with a spatula and allow the uncooked portion to flow out and cook.

8. Once the top is cooked thoroughly, add the asparagus, mushrooms and cheese, and fold into a sandwich with part of the egg.

9. Remove the omelet and cut in half. Repeat with the rest of the egg mixture.

Chapter 2: Lunchtime Recipes for Afternoon Energy

Eggs, Lox and Caramelized Onions on Bagel

Description

Afternoons do not have to be a battle with fatigue and a sluggish feeling. Allow your mid-day meal to recharge your body with fulfilling foods that bring nutrition to your organs and pep up your blood flow. You'll never miss the calories, but you will enjoy missing that afternoon slump that used to slow you down.

Yields: 4 Servings

Ingredients

4 teaspoons butter
1 sliced onion
8 eggs
2 Tablespoons heavy cream
4 ounces lox
4 toasted buns

Instructions

1. Melt 2 teaspoons butter in a skillet, add sliced onions, and cook over medium heat for 8-10 minutes, or until golden brown. Remove to a plate.

2. Beat eggs and cream in a bowl.

3. Melt remaining butter in the skillet and add mixture from bowl.

4. Add salt and pepper, to flavor, and stir constantly, until almost set.

5. Add lox and onions, stirring until heated throughout.

6. Spread on toasted bagel halves.

Silky Onion Soup

Description

Enjoy this tasty soup with a few carrot sticks and a piece of Melba toast. The creamy rich flavor will remind you of an elegant evening meal, instead of a lunch time treat.

Yields: 8 Servings

Ingredients

3 Tablespoons butter
1 sliced onion
2 garlic cloves, minced
2 leeks (white part only), cut in 1/2" strips
1 medium zucchini, sliced
½ teaspoon tarragon
¼ teaspoon salt
¼ teaspoon pepper
2 cups scallions, thinly sliced
28 ounces chicken broth
1 ½ cup water
½ cup heavy cream

Instructions

1. Melt 2 Tablespoons butter in a saucepan, over medium heat.

2. Add onion, garlic, leeks, zucchini, tarragon, salt and pepper.

3. Cover and simmer about 7 minutes
4. Stir in 1 ¾ cup scallions and cook until wilted.

5. Add broth and water and increase the heat until all is boiling.

6. Reduce heat and simmer for 10 minutes.

7. Remove from heat and break up the vegetables with a masher.

8. Return to a medium heat and add the remaining butter and the cream.

9. Heat just until boiling begins.

10. Remove from heat and sprinkle with remaining scallions.

Makes a great make ahead meal for warming up when on the run.

Tuna Salad Supreme in Tortilla Shells

Description

Give new meaning to tired tuna salad that grows old after a time or two. The right mix of veggies and a complementary bowl will turn tuna into a sought after lunch.

Yields: 4 Servings

Ingredients

4 8-inch round flour tortillas
1 Tablespoon olive oil
3 5-ounce cans Albacore tuna, drained
6 stalks celery, chopped
1 cucumber, peeled and cubed
2/3 cup mayonnaise
16 cherry tomatoes, quartered
4 lettuce leaves

Instructions

1. Heat oven to 400-degrees.

2. Take 4 oven-proof bowls and turn upside down.

3. Brush both sides of the tortillas with olive oil and place one over each bowl.

4. Bake in the oven until the tortillas are crisp and hold their shape, about 7 to 10 minutes.

5. Remove from oven and keep draped over the bowls until completely cooled.

6. In a bowl, mix the remaining ingredients (except the lettuce leaves).

7. Invert the bowls and lace each one with a lettuce leaf before adding the tuna salad.

You will never eat tuna salad on bread again!

Low-Cal Greek Salad

Description

Never miss out on the taste of feta cheese, blended perfectly in a luscious bed of romaine lettuce. Here is a great way to give in to your taste bud desires, without adding unwanted carbohydrates.

Yields: 1 Serving

Ingredients

8 leaves romaine lettuce, torn
1 cucumber, peeled and sliced
1 chopped tomato
½ cup red onion, sliced
½ cup low-fat feta cheese, crumbled
2 Tablespoons olive oil
2 Tablespoons fresh lemon juice
1 teaspoon dried oregano leaves
½ teaspoon salt

Instructions

1. Mix torn lettuce, cucumber, tomato, onion, and cheese in a large serving bowl.

2. Using a separate bowl, whisk together the oil, lemon juice, oregano, and salt.

3. Pour over salad.

Spinach Salad with Chicken and Raspberry

Description

Raspberry adds a tangy flavor to salads and chicken, so why not combine them? Adding a few other tricks will make this mid-day meal something to look forward to.

Yields: 4 Servings

Ingredients

¼ cup white vinegar
5 Tablespoons olive oil
1 teaspoon honey
½ teaspoon orange peel, shredded
½ teaspoon salt
¼ teaspoon pepper
4 skinless, boneless chicken breast halves
5 cups torn spinach
5 cups torn mixed greens
1 cup fresh raspberries
1 papaya, peeled, seeded and cubed

Instructions

1. Combine the vinegar, 4 Tablespoons olive oil, honey,

orange peel, salt and pepper.

2. Pour into an airtight jar and shake well. Store in the refrigerator to chill.

3. In a large skillet, heat over medium heat and add the remaining oil .

4. Add the chicken breasts and cook for 10 to 15 minutes, turning often, to brown all sides.

5. When no longer pink, remove from the skillet and pat out any excess oil and water.

6. Cut the warm chicken into thin strips.

7. In a large bowl, toss the greens, spinach and chicken strips.

8. Take your salad dressing and pour over the salad, tossing well.

9. Add the raspberries and cubed papaya, tossing gently.

Lettuce Roll-Ups with Pumpkin Seed Pate

Description

Move over hamburgers. This flavorful rendition of what used to be a sandwich, will make you wonder why anyone would choose meat over fresh veggies. Filled with marinated vegetables and seasoned with a unique pate, all your friends will want your recipe.

Yields: 6 Servings

Ingredients

6 large lettuce leaves

Marinated Vegetables:

2 stalks celery, sliced in 2-inch strips
1 cup carrots, shredded
¼ cup red onion, thinly sliced
2 Tablespoons flax oil
2 teaspoons lemon juice

Pate:

1 ½ garlic cloves

juice from 1 squeezed lemon

1 cup pumpkin seeds, soaked and sprouted

¼ cup flax oil

¾ teaspoon salt

¼ cup fresh parsley

¼ cup fresh basil

¼ cup dill

1/8 teaspoon turmeric

½ teaspoon fresh rosemary

Instructions for Pate

1. Using a food processor, place the garlic and pumpkins seeds inside and chop.

2. Add the lemon juice and mix until creamy.

3. Add the herbs and seasonings.

4. Pulse to finely chop all the herbs.

5. Spoon into a bowl.

Instructions for Assembly

1. Place all ingredients for marinated vegetables in a medium bowl and coat all pieces.

2. Lay flat a lettuce leaf and spread on a generous amount of pate.

3. Add ½ cup of marinated vegetables.

4. Roll up, folding the top and bottom to secure.

Chapter 3: Great Dinner Surprises

Mushroom Laced Meatballs

Description

You don't have to tell the family that they are on a low calorie diet when serving up dishes that are guaranteed to hit the spot. Lean hamburger will be anything, but boring, when dressed up with the right spices. See if anyone believes you when you admit that this dish has only 300 calories per serving.

Yields: 6 Servings

Ingredients

1 pound ground beef
1 egg
1/2 cup whole wheat bread crumbs
4 ounces shredded cheddar cheese
1/4 cup onion, chopped
1 Tablespoon Worcestershire sauce
1 Tablespoon fresh parsley, chopped

1/2 teaspoon basil

1/2 teaspoon pepper

1 Tablespoon oil

1 cup sliced mushrooms

1/2 cup beef broth

1/2 cup cooking wine

Instructions

1. Mix together meat, egg, bread crumbs, cheese, onion, Worcestershire sauce, parsley, basil and pepper.

2. Shape into 12 meatballs.

3. Add oil to skillet and brown meatballs on all sides, about 5 minutes.

4. Remove meatballs and dry on paper towels.

5. Add mushrooms to the drippings in the skillet and cook over medium heat for 2 to 3 minutes.

6. In a small bowl, mix flour, broth and wine until blended.

7. Pour over mushrooms and cook until boiling, stirring constantly.

8. Turn down heat and simmer sauce for 2 minutes.

9. Add meatballs to the creamy mixture and warm thoroughly, before serving.

Sassy Cheese and Chicken Enchiladas

Description

Kids will come running when they smell the succulent aroma of one of their favorite meals. Chicken enchiladas always top the favorites list, especially when dripping with cheese sauce. Microwave the entire meal and save time.

Yields: 6 Servings

Ingredients

2 cups cooked chicken breasts, chopped

1/2 cup chopped onion

1 garlic clove, minced

1 Tablespoon oil

4 ounces chopped green chilies

1/2 cup chicken broth

2 teaspoons chili powder

1 teaspoon cumin

4 ounces cubed cream cheese

6 6-inch flour tortillas

1/4 pound Colby or Cheddar cheese, cubed

2 Tablespoons milk

1/2 cup fresh chopped tomato

Instructions

1. In a 2-quart microwavable dish, mix onion, garlic and oil.

2. Microwave on high for 2 minutes. Stir and return for 1 more minute.

3. Remove and add chicken, chilies, broth and seasonings. Blend well.

4. Return to microwave and cook on high for 4 minutes.

5. Remove and add cream cheese, stirring until all the cheese is melted.

6. Spoon 1/2 cup of the mixture onto a tortilla shell and roll up. Repeat 6 times and place all, seam side down, on a flat microwavable dish.

7. In a clean microwavable dish, mix the Colby or Cheddar cheese, milk and 1/4 cup tomato and microwave on high for 1 minute. Stir and return for another 1 or 2 minutes.

8. Remove the cheese sauce and pour over the

enchiladas.

9. Microwave on high for 4 minutes.

10.Remove and top with remaining tomatoes.

11. Return to the microwave and cook on high for another 2 to 3 minutes.

Serve with salsa and chips.

Colorful Veggie Meatloaf

Description

Put sparkle in an old dish by using creative, and healthy vegetables. This one dish meal will add new meaning to meatloaf, as it was once known.

Yields: 8 Servings

Ingredients

1 1/2 pounds lean ground beef
3 cups white bread crumbs, toasted
1 cup diced tomatoes
1 cup fresh or frozen green beans (thawed)
1 egg
1 carrot
2 Tablespoons Worcestershire sauce
1 1/2 teaspoons salt
1/4 teaspoon pepper
1/4 cup ketchup

Instructions

1. Preheat oven to 375 degrees F
2. In a large bowl, mix all ingredients (except ketchup),

until well blended.

3. Turn into a loaf pan and top with ketchup.

4. Bake for 50 to 60 minutes, or until cooked throughout.

5. Remove and transfer to a platter, patting dry any excess fat.

Serve with a tossed salad for a filling, low calorie dinner.

Grilled Summer Kabobs

Description

Grilling during the spring and summer months can be exciting. The smell of meat that is char-broiled to perfection, can get your tummy growling. Make a delightful and low carb dinner, while including steak. A little bit goes a long way with this recipe.

Yields: 6 Servings

Ingredients

1 1/2 pounds boneless beef sirloin steak, cut into strips
1 zucchini, cut in 1-inch pieces
1 squash, cut into diagonal pieces
2 onions, quartered
12 cherry tomatoes
1/2 cup mayonnaise
1/2 cup plain yogurt
1/4 cup lemon juice
3 cloves garlic, minced
2 teaspoons minced ginger root
1/2 teaspoon cardamom
1/2 teaspoon cumin
1/2 teaspoon coriander

1/8 teaspoon red pepper

Instructions

1. Prepare the marinade by blending all seasonings, mayonnaise, yogurt and lemon juice. Put 1/2 cup of dressing aside for later.

2. Skewer the steak strips between the zucchini, squash, onions, and tomatoes.

3. Place the kabobs on a hot grill and brush with the marinade.

4. Grill for 10 or 15 minutes, or until the meat reaches the required doneness, turning and brushing twice.

5. Remove and serve with the reserved dressing.

Veggie Laced Macaroni and Cheese

Description

Macaroni and Cheese, from a box, offers little in the way of low carbs and vitamins. However, it will not take long for family to miss this simple mix of cheese and pasta. Try this homemade version that has a new twist and watch them ask for more.

Yields: 4 Servings

Ingredients

9 ounces penne noodles
1 ½ cups sharp cheddar cheese
1 Tablespoon tarragon
1/8 teaspoon ground white pepper
4 carrots, peeled and sliced
juice from one fresh orange
¼ cup water

Instructions

Warm oven to 350 degrees F.

In a saucepan, combine the carrots and juice from

orange.

Add 1/4 cup water and heat until boiling.

Turn down, cover and simmer for about 30 minutes.

Remove from heat and transfer to a blender.

Puree contents.

In a separate pan, boil the penne noodles in salted water until al dente.

Drain off the water, reserving 1 cup in the pan.

Add the drained pasta to the pan, along with the puree.

Heat on medium, stirring to coat penne.

Cook, stirring often,
Add 1 cup cheese, tarragon and white pepper.

Once the mixture becomes creamy, pour all into a greased baking dish.

Add the remaining cheese on top and bake for 20 minutes.

Remove and let stand for 5 minutes before serving.

Chapter 4: Unique Side Dishes

Fake Mashed Potatoes

Description

If your family craves meat and potatoes, this is just an old habit. However, you can give them what they want by serving a meat dish and using this unique recipe for mashed potatoes, made from fresh cauliflower. The flavor will be better, the consistency, fluffy, and that mindset of meat and potatoes will quickly dissipate.

Yields: 4 Servings

Ingredients

1 fresh cauliflower head
1 Tablespoon water
1 Tablespoon butter
2 Tablespoons heavy cream

Instructions

Chop cauliflower into small pieces and add to a large

casserole dish.

Add 1 Tablespoon water, cover, and microwave on high for 5 minutes.

Remove and let stand for 5 minute.

Drain water from cauliflower and place in a food processor.

Add butter and heavy cream.

Process until smooth.

Scoop out and place in a serving bowl.

Simplistic Green Beans

Description

Sometimes the best things in life are amazingly simple. Take this green bean dish, for example. Only two ingredients deliver taste and fulfillment, complimenting any main dish.

Yields: 4 Servings

Ingredients

1 pound fresh green beans
1 onion, cut in half and sliced thick
1 Tablespoon oil
2 Tablespoons butter
Unrefined sea salt and pepper to taste

Instructions

Using a heavy skillet, sauté green beans, over medium heat, in oil and 1 Tablespoon of butter.

Add onion pieces and continue sautéing until the onions brown.

Turn into a serving bowl and let guests season, to their liking, with salt and pepper.

Dressy Cauliflower Casserole

Description

Cauliflower is a great food for keeping carbs low, but can become quite boring when prepared over and over again. This recipe dresses up this vegetable by using other seasonings for a flavor that almost makes you forget about the main ingredient.

Yields: 6 Servings

Ingredients

1 fresh head cauliflower, broken up, or 1 16 ounce frozen bag, cooked and drained
½ cup onion, diced
1 ½ cup fresh mushrooms
2 Tablespoons butter
¼ cup heavy cream
¼ cup mayonnaise
4 ounces shredded cheddar cheese
¼ cup green onions, chopped

Instructions

Warm oven to 350 degrees F.

Place prepared cauliflower in a greased 2-quart casserole dish.

In a skillet, sauté onion and mushrooms in the butter.

Add to the cauliflower and mix.

Mix in cheese.

In a small bowl, combine cream and mayonnaise.

Pour the sauce over the cauliflower mix and coat well.

Sprinkle the top with green onions.

Bake, covered, for 25 minutes.

Remove lid and bake another 10 minutes, or until the top is brown and crispy.

Chapter 5: Fulfillment with Drinks

Pina Colada Smoothie

Description

Soft drinks and some fruit drinks can be loaded with sugar. By side-stepping this calorie boosting substance, drinks take on a more lasting flavor, keep you from tiring and give your body the liquids that they need.

Yields: 2 Servings

Ingredients

1/2 cup unsweetened coconut milk
1/4 cup plain yogurt
1/2 cup fresh pineapple chunks
1/4 teaspoon coconut extract
1 teaspoon fresh lime juice
8 ice cubes
2 packets sugar substitute
2 lime slices

Instructions

1. In a blender, add all ingredients (except lime slices).

2. Blend on high until smooth.

Add a slice of lime to the edge of each glass to add a zesty twist.

Refreshing Fruit Shake

Description

Shakes do not have to weigh you down with unhealthy calories and leaving you feel sluggish. Try this homemade version of a strawberry milkshake and forget the tired feeling. Double the recipe to share with a friend.

Yields: 1 Serving

Ingredients

1 cup strawberries
1 cup almond flavored low-fat milk
1 packet sugar substitute
1 cube tofu
1 cup ice cubes

Instructions

1. Blend together strawberries, milk, sugar substitute, and tofu in a blender.

2. Add ice cubes and blend again.

Awesome Juice Spritzer

Description

Keeping the kids (and adults) away from soft drinks can be a never ending chore. Keep a 2-liter bottle of refreshing juice spritzer in the frig and no one will even miss the pop.

Yields: 6 Servings

Ingredients

9 ounces pineapple, orange, or pomegranate juice
48 ounces club soda or sparkling water

Instructions

1. Add juice to club soda or sparkling water, using a 2 liter air tight bottle.

Freshly processed and strained fruit can also be used in the place of juice.

Honey Dew Smoothie

Description

Add variety to your beverages by using a little thought of ingredient. The flavor will bring a new twist to boring fruit juices. Light and healthy, this drink only has 110 calories per serving. Increase ingredients to share with family and friends.

Yields: 2 Servings

Ingredients

4 cups cubed honey dew
2 apples, peeled, cored and cubed
2 kiwi fruits, peeled and sliced
3 packets sugar substitute
2 Tablespoons lemon juice
2 cups ice cubes

Instructions

1. Combine all ingredients (except ice cubes) in a blender and blend well.

2. Add ice cubes and blend until ice becomes broken

into small pieces.

Apricot Peach Slush

Description

This fruity drink has become a favorite of diabetics because of the sweet flavor and smooth texture. It's hard to think that something so refreshing can be good for you, but it is. Keep plenty of apricot nectar on hand because this beverage will go fast.

Yields: 6 Servings

Ingredients

15 ½ ounces apricot nectar, chilled
2 fresh peaches, peeled, pitted and sliced
1 ½ cups crushed ice
1 Tablespoon lemon juice
1 ½ cups chilled carbonated water

Instructions

1. In a blender, combine the apricot nectar, peaches, lemon juice and crushed ice.

2. Blend until smooth.

3. Spoon into a tall glass, filling halfway.

4. Fill the glass to the top with carbonated water.

Smooth Strawberry Passion

Description

Forget the milkshakes and all the calories and instead, make up a batch of Smooth Strawberry Passion drinks. Low in carbs and fat, this drink is great for a gathering or just to sit on the porch on a hot summer day.

Yields: 6 Servings

Ingredients

4 cups fresh strawberries, sliced
1 banana
1 kiwi fruit
16 ounces vanilla yogurt
1 cup ice cubes

Instructions

Using a blender, add strawberries, banana, and yogurt.

Blend until creamy.

Add ice cubes, one at a time, blending until they are broken up.

Pour in glasses, garnishing with kiwi fruit.

Wean Off of Soft Drinks

In a world of perfection, you would cut out all soda. The sugary sweeteners, found in soda, is almost impossible to break down. However, the addiction to soft drinks can cause you to abandon a new eating plan, after a day or two. If you currently have sugary soda in your daily life, definitely change to a diet brand - but don't try to cut it out cold turkey. You want to succeed in your new diet, so it is okay to start out slow. Slowly wean yourself off of the addictive, artificial taste by trading for a more refreshing taste of natural ingredients.

Chapter 6: Make Ahead Snacks

Sweet Popcorn Extravaganza

Description

Showtime in front of the TV will become even more exciting when there is a big bowl of crunchy, sweet snacks ready for each turn. Make this light and wholesome finger food ahead of time and keep in an air tight container.

Yields: 8 Servings

Ingredients

4 Tablespoons butter, melted
2 egg whites
2 packets sugar substitute
½ teaspoon vanilla extract
½ teaspoon cinnamon
¼ teaspoon salt
1 ½ cups low-carb cereal flakes
3 ounces pecans or almonds
4 cups pop corn

Instructions

1. Heat oven to 300 degrees F.

2. Lay a sheet of aluminum foil over a baking sheet and spray with Canola oil.

3. In a small bowl, combine butter, egg whites, sugar substitute, vanilla, cinnamon and salt.

4. Whisk the egg mixture until well blended.

5. Using a large bowl, add cereal and nuts and coat with the melted butter.

6. Add popcorn and lightly toss.

7. Pour mixture onto the baking sheet and spread evenly.

8. Bake for 20 to 25 minutes, or until crispy.

9. Remove and cool.

Store in an air tight container until show time. By adding the popcorn to the mixture last, there will be less clumps for hands to grab.

Granola Mini Balls

Description

These little bundles are the perfect size for snacking or grabbing as a quick energy picker-upper. Leave a plateful on the table and the refrigerator door will have less activity.

Yields: 6 Servings

Ingredients

2 cups granola
½ cup raisins
½ cup pecans, chopped
½ cup dried apricots
1 cup low-fat dried milk
1 cup creamy peanut butter
1/3 cup honey

Instructions

1. In a large bowl, mix granola, raisins, pecans, apricots, dried milk, and honey.

2. Gradually add peanut butter, stirring until all

ingredients are well covered.

3. Using your hands, form into small balls and place on small squares of waxed paper.

4. Place the balls, including the waxed paper on a serving plate. The waxed paper will keep the balls from sticking to one another.

Homemade Sweet Granola Mix

Description

Teach your kids how to have a great snack by letting them help make this sweet, crunchy treat. They will learn how to eat healthier, plus have something to munch on while playing video games.

Yields: 8 Servings

Ingredients

1 cup rolled oats
1 cup almonds
1 cup unsalted peanuts
1 cup raw sunflower seeds
1 cup flax seeds
1 cup sweetened coconut flakes
1 cup dried cranberries
3 Tablespoons brown sugar syrup

Instructions

1. Preheat oven to 250 degrees F.

2. Line a baking sheet with parchment sheets.

3. Use a large mixing bowl and add all ingredients.

4. Mix well with a wooden spoon or spatula.

5. Spread onto the baking sheet and flatten.

6. Bake for 15 minutes.

7. Remove and break up the granola pieces.

8. Bake for an additional 15 minutes.

9. Remove and cool.

10. Place into an airtight container.

Healthy Workout Granola Mix

Description

Here is another type of granola treat that is favored by athletes after a good workout. However, it was soon found to be a favorite of youngsters, as well.

Yields: 8 servings

Ingredients

1 cup rolled oats
1 cup almonds
1 cup dried cranberries
1 ½ cups butter
½ cup brown sugar
2 Tablespoons honey
½ teaspoon vanilla extract

Instructions

1. Preheat oven to 375 degrees F.

2. Coat baking tray with spray canola oil
3. In a large bowl, combine the oats, almonds, dried cranberries, and ground cinnamon.

4. Blend well with a large wooden spoon or spatula.

5. Add the butter, brown sugar, honey and vanilla extract together in a separate bowl, blending well.

6. Pour the butter mixture into the dry ingredients and mix until all is coated.

7. Spread the mixture onto the greased baking tray and press down to flatten.

8. Place in the oven for 20 to 25 minutes.

9. Remove and cool.

10. Either cut into bars, or break up the pieces for a bite size treat.

Low-Carb Nachos and Fixings

Description

Many people admit that their toughest part of staying on a low-carb diet, is giving up chips. Here is a unique way to have it all. Chips, cheese, salsa, at an amazing 6.5 net carbs. The secret is in the chips and here is a way to have your cake and eat it, too.

Yields: 10 Servings

Ingredients

8 ounces low-carb soy chips
1 cup chopped black olives
4 ½ ounces chopped, mild green chilies
12 ounces cheddar cheese, grated
2/3 cup sour cream
2/3 cup salsa

Instructions

1. Move rack in oven to within 6 inches of the broiler and preheat to broil.

2. Line 2 baking sheets with aluminum foil and spray

lightly, with canola oil spray.

3. Arrange the soy chips on the baking sheets in a single layer.

4. Top each chip with olives and chilies.

5. Sprinkle with cheese.

6. Place in oven and broil for 45 to 60 seconds.

7. Remove and transfer to a platter.

8. Place sour cream in one small bowl and the salsa in another.

9. Serve together.

Crispy Fried Fish with Lemon Sauce

Description

Who says you can't have fried fish on a low-carb diet? Choose pollock, whiting, haddock or scrod, and don't forget the sauce.

Yields: 4 Servings

Ingredients

4 8-ounce fish fillets
1 egg
2 ounces baked potato chips, ground
2 Tablespoons water
2 Tablespoons canola oil
½ cup mayonnaise
3 Tablespoons fresh dill, chopped
2 teaspoons lemon zest, grated
¼ teaspoon pepper

Instructions

1. Spread chip crumbs on a flat surface lined with waxed paper.

2. In a wide bowl, whisk 1 egg with water and brush on each fillet.

3. Heat a non-stick skillet to medium heat and add 1 Tablespoon canola oil
4. Dredge each fillet through the crumbs and place in the hot skillet.

5. Turn each fillet once after cooking about 3 to 4 minutes, or until golden brown.

6. Gently remove to plates
7. In a small bowl, mix the mayonnaise, dill, zest and pepper for dip.

Chapter 7: Let's Have a Picnic

Oriental Cabbage Salad

Description

Summer comes with lots of potlucks and bar-b-ques. Trying to watch your eating habits can be very trying with hamburgers and hot dogs being served. Start bringing great side dishes to get togethers and introduce the crowd to great tasting foods.

Yields: 4 Servings

Ingredients

½ head grated, green cabbage
3 chopped scallions
2 Tablespoons sesame oil
2 Tablespoons rice wine vinegar
2 Tablespoons toasted sesame seeds

Instructions

1. In a large serving bowl, combine the cabbage,

scallions, oil and vinegar.

2. Toss well, then refrigerate.

3. Right before serving, add the sesame seeds and toss lightly.

Kickin' Deviled Eggs

Description

Deviled eggs are an all-time favorite at picnics, but these beauties will make the crowd stop and say, WOW! The special ingredient may surprise you, and certainly, anyone who indulges. With 1 gram of carbs and 178 calories, maybe it won't hurt to have a couple.

Yields: 20 eggs

Ingredients

10 large eggs
4 Tablespoons cream cheese
½ cup mayonnaise
2 Tablespoons fresh chives, minced
2 teaspoons wasabi paste
pepper
1 teaspoon sea salt

Instructions

1. Boil eggs in a single layer, using a large saucepan, for 7 minutes.

2. Turn off heat and cover saucepan for 15 minutes.

3. Drain water off and refill with cold water. Let stand for at least 10 minutes.

4. Peel eggs and cut in half, long way.

5. Remove yolks and place in a large bowl.

6. Add the cream cheese and wasabi paste.

7. Mash with a fork or masher until everything is blended and resembles small crumbs.

8. Stir in the mayonnaise and chives and add pepper to taste.

9. Place the yolk mixture in a pastry bag and squeeze filling into the white cups of the eggs.

10. Make a swirling motion, beginning with the outer layer and working to a point in the middle.

11. Just before serving, sprinkle with sea salt.

Chicken Waldorf Salad

Description

Everyone loves the flavor of apples and walnuts, mixed with greens and a tart dressing. Make it a meal by adding chicken and using a new kind of dressing that will make guests request, time and time again.

Yields: 4 Servings

Ingredients

4 cooked and cubed chicken breasts
1 cup chopped celery
1 ½ cup chopped apples
4 ounces walnut pieces
4 Tablespoons raisins
1 cup low-fat Italian dressing
10 cups Iceberg and Bibb lettuce

Instructions

1. Place the lettuce, chicken, apples and celery in a large serving bowl and toss well.

2. Pour the Italian dressing over all and toss to coat.

3. Add the walnut pieces and raisins, gently blending.

Fresh Green Bean and Tomato Italiano

Description

There is nothing more flavorful than the taste of fresh green beans that are served up steamed and crunchy. Bring this dish to your outdoor party and you will find that even the youngsters will be tempted with their presence. This is a quick and easy side dish that delivers a compliment to any type of meat.

Yields: 6 Servings

Ingredients

3 cups fresh green beans
2 plum tomatoes, sliced into thin wedges
2 Tablespoons fresh basil
¼ cup Italian dressing

Instructions

1. Steam green beans for 10 minutes, just long enough to remove the raw texture.

2. Cool and add tomatoes and basil.

3. Pour dressing over all and toss lightly, just to coat.

Confetti Pasta Salad

Description

Here is a dish that is almost too beautiful to eat. Colorful and robust, it will seem more like a main dish than a complimentary side. Increase the size to share for an outdoor BBQ or other picnic event.

Yields: 4 Servings

Ingredients

1 cup multicolored, low-carb penne, cooked
4 artichoke hearts, diced
4 ounces thinly sliced turkey breast strips
8 ounces fresh mozzarella, diced
4 Tablespoon red pepper
8 Tablespoons fresh, chopped green beans
4 Tablespoons olive oil
4 teaspoons balsamic vinegar
2 teaspoons fresh oregano, chopped

Instructions

1. Combine pasta, artichoke hearts, turkey, mozzarella, red pepper and green beans in a large salad bowl.

2. In a small bowl, mix oil, vinegar, and oregano.

3. Pour over the pasta mixture and toss.

Cobb Salad with Crab

Description

Seafood is the main ingredient that gives this salad a wonderful flavor. Along with other cobb salad favorite additions, this side dish goes very well with those lake-caught fish.

Yields: 4 Servings

Ingredients

12 cups romaine lettuce, torn into bite-size pieces
12 ounce cooked crab meat
2 cups cherry tomatoes, halved
1 cup crumbled blue cheese
½ cup olive oil raspberry flavored dressing

Instructions

1. In a large serving bowl, add lettuce, crab meat, tomatoes and blue cheese.

2. Toss well then add dressing and toss again.

Chapter 8: Exciting Desserts

Chocolate Sponge Cake with Strawberries

Description

There is something wrong with a low-carb diet that does not allow for the sweet pleasures in life, mainly cake and chocolate. This dessert will satisfy both with rich flavor and texture.

Yields: 10 Servings

Ingredients

7 egg whites
1/8 tsp cream of tartar
¾ cup sugar
3 egg yolks
1 teaspoon vanilla
1 cup cake flour
3 Tablespoons melted butter
1 ½ ounces semisweet chocolate
2 Tablespoons canola oil
12 plump strawberries

Instructions

1. Heat oven to 350 degr F.

2. Use a large bowl to beat the egg whites and cream of tartar until foamy.

3. Add the sugar, gradually, while whipping into a meringue, with soft peaks.

4. In another bowl, beat together the egg yolks and vanilla.

5. Add the egg yolk mixture to the egg whites, gradually, folding until well blended.

6. Fold in the flour, stirring until all has been absorbed.

7. Pour batter into the cake batter and fold gently.

9. Spoon the batter into a 10-inch tube pan and bake for 35-40 minutes, or until the center proves clean, with a tooth pick.

10. Remove the cake and turn upside down on a large bottle so all sides are exposed to the air.

11. Cool for about an hour.

12. Remove the pan and run a knife along the sides of the pan to loosen the cake, then invert onto a wire rack to further cool.

13. Place on a serving dish.

14. Melt the chocolate and oil, slowly to keep from scorching and drizzle over the cooled cake.

15. Dot the top with strawberries.

Luscious Lime Cheesecake Tarts

Description

Cheesecake can add the final touch to a great meal, or be a special treat for friends that visit. Adding the tartness of lime and the sweetness of kiwi, will let you savor every bite.

Yields: 12 Servings

Ingredients

12 vanilla wafers
¾ cup cottage cheese
8 ounces low-fat cream cheese
¼ cup sugar or sugar substitute
2 eggs
1 Tablespoon grated lime rind
1 Tablespoon fresh lime juice
1 teaspoon vanilla
¼ cup vanilla flavored yogurt
2 kiwis, peeled, sliced and halved

Instructions

1. Using a 12-cup muffin pan, line each cup with a paper

muffin liner.

2. Heat oven to 350 degrees F.

3. Place a vanilla wafer in the bottom of each cup.

4. Using a blender, add the cottage cheese, cream cheese and sugar. Blend well.

5. Add the eggs, lime rind, lime juice and vanilla. Beat until smooth.

6. Spoon the mixture into the lined muffin cups and bake for 15-20 minutes, or until well set.

7. Remove from oven and chill completely.

8. Right before serving, spread the vanilla flavored yogurt on top and garnish with kiwi pieces.

Fruity Bread Pudding

Description

Bread pudding can become a sinful dish when laced with peaches and cream. Serve up this delightful dessert to family and friends. Have the recipe ready to share because everyone will want to know your secret ingredients.

Yields: 12 Servings

Ingredients

1 teaspoon butter, softened
6 slices low-carb bread, cubed
1 ½ cups fresh or frozen chopped peaches
4 eggs
1 cup heavy cream
½ cup sugar
¼ teaspoon nutmeg
1 ½ teaspoons vanilla
2 Tablespoons sliced almonds

Instructions

1. Warm oven to 350 F degrees.

2. Butter an 8-inch square baking dish

3. Add bread crumbs and peaches to dish and toss.

4. In a medium-sized bowl, add eggs, cream, sugar, nutmeg and vanilla, and whisk together.

5. Pour the egg mixture over the bread and peaches.

6. Let stand for 10 minutes to allow the bread to absorb the liquid mixture.

7. Sprinkle almonds on top of the dish.

8. Place the dish inside a 9x11 pan, filled with boiling water. The water should rise halfway up the sides of the 8-inch dish.

9. Bake for 45 to 50 minutes, or until a clean knife shows that it is done.

Almond Ricotta Pudding

Description

Take a break with a smooth, luscious pudding that is satisfying and only 8 carbs per serving. Quick to make, this recipe is designed for 1 serving but can be stretched to include the whole family.

Yields: 1 Serving

Ingredients

½ cup ricotta cheese
¼ teaspoon almond extract
1 packet sweetener
1 teaspoon slivered toasted almonds

Instructions

1. Mix the ricotta cheese, almond extract and sugar substitute.

2. Sprinkle with almonds.

Enjoy.

Heavenly Chocolate Sorbet

Description

Remember the fudge ice pops that you enjoyed as a child? Here is an adult version that will bring back memories, yet satisfy the grown up you. You will need an ice-cream maker for this recipe. This treat is not for kids, the more reason to sneak away and enjoy.

Yields: 4 Servings

Ingredients

2 cups ice cold water
1 teaspoon unflavored gelatin
1 ½ cups sugar-free chocolate syrup
1 cup low-fat milk
3 Tablespoons dark rum

Instructions

1. Add 2 Tablespoons ice water in a glass measuring cup.

2. Sprinkle with gelatin.

3. Microwave for 20 seconds to dissolve the gelatin.

3. In a medium-sized bowl, add ¾ cup syrup, the remaining ice water, milk and rum.

4. Stir until blended.

5. Add the remaining chocolate syrup into the mix and whisk.

6. Add the dissolved gelatin and stir.

7. Pour the mixture into an ice-cream maker and churn, according to instructions.

8. Remove and place in an airtight container and place in the freezer until ready to serve.

Non Traditional Squash Pie

Description

Pumpkin pie may be the tradition, but there's a new version in town. Serve up this wonderful dessert that offers much lower calories and carbs and start a new traditional during the holidays, or any time.

Yields: 8 Servings

Ingredients

3 cups cooked winter squash, mashed
¾ cup unsweetened coconut milk
¼ cup honey
3 eggs
2 teaspoons pumpkin pie spice
1 ½ teaspoons maple extract
1 ½ Tablespoons arrowroot powder
1 ¼ teaspoons unrefined sea salt, finely ground
½ teaspoon sugar

Instructions

1. Warm oven to 350 degr F.

2. Mix all ingredients with a mixer or in a food processor. If the consistency is too thick, add a little water, 1 teaspoon each, until no longer stiff.

3. Pour into a greased 10-inch pie pan and bake for 50 to 60 minutes, or until a knife comes out clean, when placed in the center.

4. Allow pie to cool then chill for another 30 minutes, to firm.

Chapter 9: Wise Wok Cooking

Shrimp Egg Rolls

Description

Reintroduce your wok to keep fat and sugar limited. It may take some time to prepare these awesome egg rolls, but the results are well worth the trouble.

Yields: 8 Servings

Ingredients

½ pounds raw shrimp, cleaned and deveined

1 teaspoon sherry

1 teaspoon salt

½ teaspoon cornstarch

3 Tablespoons canola oil

3 cups diced celery

½ teaspoon sugar

1 Tablespoon water

½ cup fresh bean sprouts

1 cup shredded lettuce

1 cup chopped water chestnuts

16 egg-roll wrappers

Instructions

1. In a small bowl, combine shrimp, sherry, salt and cornstarch.

2. Let the mixture marinate for 12 to minutes.

3. Heat 1 tablespoon oil in work.

4. Add shrimp mixture and stir-fry until shrimp is pink and firm.

5. Remove to a mixing bowl.

6. Add remaining oil to wok and add celery, stir-frying for 2 to 3 minutes.

7. Add sugar and water.

8. Cover and let steam for 1 minute.

9. Remove cover and stir-fry until all the liquid has evaporated.

10. Add to shrimp mixture.

11. Add remaining ingredients.

12. Blend well.

13. Prepare wrappers by laying out flat.

14. Fill each one with ¼ cup shrimp mixture.

15. Lift lower triangle of wrapper over filling and tuck the point under.

16. Leave the upper point of the wrapper flat.

17. Bring the 2 end flaps up and over the enclosed filling and press flaps down firmly.

18. Brush cold water over the exposed triangles and roll the filled portion until you have a neat package. The water will seal your ingredients protectively.

19. Repeat until you have 16 filled egg rolls.

20. Fill the wok with 3 inches of oil in the center.

21. Heat to 375 degrees F.

22. Using tongs, lower 4 eggs rolls into the oil and deep fry for 3 to 4 minutes, or until golden brown.

23. Drain on paper towels, blotting out all of the oil.

24. Repeat until all egg rolls have been cooked.

Serve with hot mustard, plum sauce or soy sauce. You can also store for later use by cooling and wrapping in plastic wrap, then placing in freezer bags to refrigerate or freeze.

Mandarin Cauliflower and Broccoli Medley

Description

Making your vegetables more interesting, will create a reason for your family to try any new variation. The aroma of this mixture, while stir-frying, will have everyone sitting at the table, ready to enjoy.

Yields: 4 Servings

Ingredients

2 Tablespoons canola oil
½ teaspoon salt
10 mushrooms, sliced lengthwise
1 small onion, minced
1 cup water
1 ½ cups bite-size cauliflower pieces
1 ½ cups bite-size broccoli pieces
½ cup water
2 teaspoons sugar
2 teaspoons cornstarch dissolved in 1 Tablespoon water

Instructions

1. Heat oil and salt in wok.

2. Add mushrooms and onion.

3. Stir-fry for 2 minutes or until tender.

4. Add water and bring to a boil.

5. Cover and steam for 5 minutes.

6. Uncover and add broccoli.

7. Cover and steam for an additional 10 minutes, stirring occasionally.

8. Uncover and add remaining water and sugar.

9. Bring to a simmer and add cornstarch mix.

10. Stir until sauce thickens and all vegetables are well coated.

Stir Fry Chicken and Peaches

Description

A delicate sauce make this stir fry chicken recipe a hit with the family. Low-cal and nutritious, peaches all extra flavor to a classic sweet and sour classic dish.

Yields: 6 to 8 Servings

Ingredients

1 3-pound chicken, cut into 8 pieces
1 teaspoon salt
½ teaspoon poultry seasoning
3 Tablespoons cornstarch
1 cup canola oil plus 1 Tablespoon oil
1 clove garlic, peeled and crushed
8 ounces frozen sliced, unsweetened peaches, thawed
1 Tablespoon sugar
2 Tablespoons lemon juice
½ cup chicken broth
2 teaspoons cornstarch dissolved in 1 Tablespoon water
10 ounces frozen snow peas
3 cups hot cooked rice

Instructions

1. Fill wok half full with water.

2. Place chicken pieces in a shallow baking dish and sprinkle with salt and poultry seasoning.

3. Place dish on a wire rack atop the wok and cover.

4. Cover chicken and turn wok on medium-high.

5. Steam the chicken for 45 minutes.

6. Remove and dry chicken pieces.

7. Rub cornstarch into each chicken piece.

8. Remove water from wok and wipe dry.

9. Add 1 cup canola oil into wok and heat to just under sizzling.

10. Fry chicken pieces in the hot oil, 2 or 3 pieces at a time until lightly browned.

11. Remove to a plate, lined with paper towels.

12. Pour oil out of wok and discard.

13. Add 1 Tablespoon oil to wok, add garlic, and stir-fry until brown.

14. Remove and discard garlic.

15. Add peaches and sugar, snow peas, stirring into the garlic liquid.

16. Stir in lemon juice.

17. Add chicken broth and heat to boiling.

18. Stir in dissolved cornstarch.

19. Add snow peas, stirring into the liquid.

20. Cover and steam for 30 seconds.

21. Add chicken pieces to wok and cover.

22. Steam for 30 seconds or until chicken is heated.

Serve over hot cooked rice.

Oriental Rice

Description

It seems that every time you have a Chinese-type of meal, there is tons of white rice left over. Put it to good use with this tasty oriental rice recipe. It will make a great side dish for a lunch or dinner menu

Yields: 4 to 6 Serving

Ingredients

1 Tablespoon oil
2 cups cold cooked rice
½ cup chopped water chestnuts
½ cup raisins
¼ cup soy sauce

Instructions

1. Heat oil in wok.

2. Add rice and cook, stirring until coated with oil.

3. Add water chestnuts and raisins.

4. Stir-fry until all is heated.

5. Add soy sauce and blend well.

6. Turn into a serving bowl.

Small portions of leftover meat can also be used for additional flavor.

Sweet and Sour Shrimp

Description

Who doesn't love the awesome flavor of sweet and sour sauce, mixed with shrimp and fresh vegetables. Here is a recipe that will amaze your taste buds and satisfy your hunger.

Yields: 4 Servings

Ingredients

1 carrot, peeled and diagonally sliced
1 green pepper, cut into 1-inch squares
2 cups canola oil
½ teaspoon salt
8 ounces breaded, frozen shrimp
1 clove garlic, peeled and flattened
1 cup unsweetened pineapple chunks, drained (save the juice)
¾ cup mixed sweet pickles, drained

Sauce Ingredients

1 ¼ cup unsweetened pineapple juice
¼ cup white wine vinegar

1 Tablespoon soy sauce

1/3 cup brown sugar

1/4 cup catsup

2 Tablespoons cornstarch

Instructions

Prepare the Sweet and Sour Sauce first.

1. In a small saucepan, combine 1 cup pineapple juice, vinegar, soy sauce, sugar and catsup.

2. Stir over medium heat until simmering.

3. Dissolve cornstarch in ¼ cup pineapple juice and add to pan.

4. Stir until smooth.

5. Remove from heat and set aside.

Stir-Fry Section

1. Place carrot slices in saucepan and cover with water.

2. Boil for 5 minutes

3. Add green pepper and boil for another 5 minutes.

4. Drain and set aside.

5. Add oil and salt to wok.

6. Heat to 375 degrees F.

7. Fry the frozen shrimp, a few at a time, until lightly browned.

8. Drain on paper towels.

9. Remove oil from wok and wipe clean with paper towels.

10. Discard oil.

11. Add 1 Tablespoon oil to wok.

12. Set to high heat.

13. Add garlic, rubbing against sides and bottom until lightly browned.

14. Remove and discard.

15. Add peppers and carrots.

16. Stir-fry for 30 seconds.

17. Add the sweet and sour sauce.

18. Next, add the pineapple chunks and pickles.

19. Stir-fry until hot.

20. Add cooked shrimp and cover all with sauce.

21. Spoon over hot cooked rice.

Pears Cardinal

Description

No one will find these pears boring with the succulent flavor of raspberries, surrounding them. Easy to make while you have your wok out, or use your stove top. Attractive, rich and melt-in-your mouth consistency, make this dessert a great finish to any meal.

Yields: 8 to 10 Servings

Ingredients

6 ripe pears
Red food coloring
20 ounces frozen raspberries, thawed (or fresh is even better)
2 Tablespoons sugar
2 teaspoons cornstarch, dissolved in 2 Tablespoons water
¼ cup kirsch liqueur, or raspberry flavored syrup

Instructions

1. Place a rack in wok that is filled with simmering water.

2. Stand up pears on the rack and cover.

3. Steam for 10 to 15 minutes.

4. Remove pears from rack.

5. Run under cold water to gently remove skin.

6. Rub each pear with a little red food coloring for a blushed appearance.

7. Refrigerate until chilled.

8. Blend raspberries in a blender.

9. Strain out seeds.

10. Place the raspberry puree in a saucepan and bring to a boil.

11. Stir in sugar and dissolved cornstarch.

12. Keep stirring until mixture thickens.

13. Remove from heat and add liqueur or flavored syrup.

14. Refrigerate until well chilled.

15. When ready to serve, place on pear in a serving dish and spoon the sauce over the top.

Chapter 10: List of Low-Carb Foods

Trying to keep all of the terms straight, like carbohydrates, calories, low-fat, and induction, can be difficult to understand. Not all low-carb foods are low-fat, or low in calories. Start with this list of foods that can keep anyone on the straight and narrow in beginning a low-carb diet. After a while, you will learn, just by tasting, how some foods dull your palate in enjoying the rich flavor of natural foods. One of these is sugar. It is a known fact that refined sugar decreases your ability to savor flavor. By ridding your diet of refined sugar, bleached white flour, margarine, and other processed, synthetic additives, you will begin to enjoy the wholesome flavor that low-carb natural foods have to offer.

- Cucumbers
- Broccoli
- Iceberg Lettuce
- Celery
- White Mushrooms
- Turnips
- Radishes
- Romaine Lettuce

- Asparagus
- Green Pepper
- Okra
- Cauliflower
- Cabbage
- Red Bell Pepper
- Spinach
- Beets
- Green Beans
- Carrots
- Kale
- Sugar Snap Peas
- Corn
- Onions
- Watermelon
- Strawberries
- Cantaloupe
- Avocado
- Blackberries
- Honeydew Melon
- Grapefruit
- Oranges
- Peaches
- Papaya
- Cranberries
- Plums
- Raspberries
- Pineapple
- Nectarine
- Blueberries

- Apples
- Pears
- Kiwi Fruit
- Cherries
- Tangerines
- Mango

If you feel that you just can't stay away from refined sugar, try these natural alternatives in cooking and see how quickly your habit begins to fade.

- Molasses
- Sorghum
- Real Maple Syrup
- Maple Sugar
- Sucanat or Rapadura
- Agave Syrup
- Coconut Sugar
- Honey

Bread is a real obstacle for many that have grown up on products made from white flour. If you are able to find bread products with any of the following main ingredients, you will be doing your body a favor.

- Corn
- Soybeans
- Oat Bran
- Barley

- Organic Sprouted Wheat
- Millet

Pasta has grown popular in making quick meals but the ingredients can be full of carbs. While many companies are slow to transform a popular-selling product into one that offers good nutrition, one company is gaining ground because of the low-carb content. Known as Shirataki, the starch is made from the root of devil's tongue, a type of yam. While you will probably never find this product in your local grocery store, keep your eyes open for new types of pasta alternatives in the foreign cuisine section.

Chapter 11: Tips for Prepping

People raised in countries, outside of the United States, are constantly amazed at how our grocery shopping is done. They are used to shopping for fresh produce and seafood on a daily basis, not weekly, as is practiced in the states. How can anything be fresh when it is allowed to set for a week?

To say that it is simple to eat healthier on a low carb diet, according to American standards, would be misleading. Manufacturers of ready-made food stuffs , count on the fact that there is too little time to spend on healthy eating. Popping a cardboard box into the microwave or opening a can, has replaced wholesome foods with convenience. Unfortunately, this way of thinking has led us to where we are today. Weight gain, inadequate vitamin supply, and slow metabolism, is the result of pumping your body with preservatives and sugars that prevent a healthy system. While time is on everyone's mind, there are some short cuts that you can take to prepare for low carb meals.

Freeze, Freeze, Freeze

In the summer, fresh vegetables are everywhere. But

when winter sets in, finding produce can make your search for fresh foods, a real chore. This year, snap up those great looking veggies and freeze so you will have plenty on hand during the winter months.

Not all vegetables freeze well. Those with a high water content can become mushy and less flavorful, like onions and cucumbers. But many other types can retain their shape, presence and vitamins, for meal prepping. Here are some examples of vegetables that can be frozen and ready to use:

- Asparagus
- Beans
- Broccoli
- Cauliflower
- Squash and Zucchini
- Eggplant
- Snow Peas

How to Properly Freeze:

It is not difficult to prepare vegetables for future use, but it does take a little bit of planning. Pick a day for putting up your family's favorite veggies and follow these simple instructions to make an ample supply.

Supplies needed:

- 3-quart Saucepan
- Wire Basket
- Jelly roll pan
- Waxed paper
- Freezer Bags
- Marking Pen

Instructions for Blanching

Select your veggies and prepare by cleaning, cutting and making meal ready.

Fill the saucepan half full of water and bring to a boil.

Put the prepared veggies into the wire basket and plunge into the boiling water for 3 minutes.

Remove and drain. Pat dry to remove any excess water.

Line the jelly roll pan with waxed paper and lay out your vegetables in single file.

Place the jelly roll pan in the freezer, just long enough for the food to freeze.

Remove and place in freezer bags, squeezing out as much excess water, as possible.

Mark and date each bag and return to the freezer.

By getting into the habit of preparing garden fresh vegetables for future use, you can rest assured that your family will receive no preservatives or additives from packaged foods.

10 Tips for Staying on a Low-Cal Plan

No one claims that it is easy to break bad habits, but if you look at where you are, and where you want to be, anything is possible. Remember when you thought that using a cell phone was the most impossible thing you had ever done? But now you probably wonder how you ever lived without it. Everyone dislikes change but when the future turns out for the better, you wonder how you ever thought differently. Try some of these tips and you will soon be forgetting about those bad eating habits.

1. Use coconut as a sweetener. Why is coconut downplayed so much? It is a wonderful, sweet and tasty type of low-carb accessory that can become irreplaceable. Use it in main dish recipes, savor the juice and discover that it is very addicting.

2. Who started the rumor that eggs were bad? Eggs are

a great source of protein and can be eaten alone or used in salads and meals. They are also very portable for a quick energy boost. Use to make sauces, to add texture to foods, or just as a snack in the middle of the day.

3. Never throw leftovers away. You just spent a lot of time on a low-cal meal for your family and believe it or not, you have some scraps to deal with. You already know how good they are for you so wrap them up and use on a salad for lunch tomorrow.

4. Herbs are better than salt. We all have the habit of salting everything that is set in front of us. Break this habit by keeping a variety of herbs close by. The selection will be interesting and fun, plus a lot better than salt, which does nothing but harm your body.

5. Rice is a great filler but not the best when it comes to nutrition. Try something different, like ground cauliflower. The taste will not be so ho-hum and you might just trick your brain into thinking that it is rice, but somehow, even better.

6. Make good use of your muffin pan. Part of the problem with staying on a low- carb diet menu, is thinking that you are going to starve. The portions seem so tiny and your mind just cannot grab hold of the fact

that you will ever be satisfied. Start using a muffin pan to fill with portions so you will get used to having enough. Start with something filling, like pudding or chicken salad. You will be surprised just how much a muffin cup can hold.

7. Salads can be the spice of life. How many other foods are so flexible to accept fruit, meat, and vegetables, without ruining the taste? In addition, dressings and sauces can be an endless supply of flavor. From cheeses to herbs, lemons and limes, you can transform a salad into any flavor you desire.

8. Think of a lettuce leaf as a piece of bread and the need to be fulfilled with a sandwich, will slowly fade away. Wraps are becoming popular with anything and everything. Meat, cheese, pickles, or a mixture of favorite foods. Iceberg lettuce has big meaty leaves for wrapping up tuna salad, eggs, chicken breast, and more.

9. Go on an adventure to an Asian store and look at the labels of pasta. You will probably see some words that are foreign to you, but more than likely, they represent roots and vegetables instead of chemical additives that you do recognize. Asians are not big on bread and grains that make them feel sluggish. Ask someone in the market about the ingredients, or write down the names

and search for yourself.

10. If sweets are your downfall, don't deprive yourself and make the craving worse. Enjoy some chocolate or puddings that can be found on a low carb diet food list. Make ahead to keep on hand for when that craving hits.

Deciding to go on a low-carb diet is not just a choice for losing weight, but changing the way that you look at food. Our society has become accustomed to eating anything that announces 'low-fat' or 'low-carb, that we have been brainwashed into accepting almost anything. Always shop for fresh, or frozen, and learn to enjoy the taste of food that has been replaced with high fat and glucose filled preservatives. Not only will you feel better, but your weight will automatically begin to burn off and give you more energy.

Section 2: Paleolithic Cookbook

The standard western diet may be hurting or killing your body in so many ways, that it can be difficult to keep up with all of the health reports related to unhealthy eating. The Paleolithic diet has been popularly known for many decades, however history seems to show that early human ancestors were living on this "diet" was around 200,000 years ago! Humans were introduced into farming approximately 10,000 years producing a heavy growth grains, bread, pasta, starchy foods and processed foods. However, evidence suggests that evolution is slow to adapt to new types of food that the body may not be used to. This is why the foods including (modern) bread, grease, and processed foods are hard for humans to move on from and onto a healthier lifestyle.

What is Paleo?

The paleo lifestyle tries to follow the diet of those from ancient times of indigenous people and is referred to as the "Paleolithic Diet" as it is from the Stone Age or Paleolithic Age era. The paleolithic diet has additional names it is referred to including, "Stone Age Diet", "Hunter-Gatherer Diet", or the "Cave Man Diet". The Paleolithic diet offers a plethora of health benefits for those who have given it a try. The paleolithic diet isn't another fad diet as it has been a way of eating thousands of years and it is a healthier option for people to take. Anthropologists have found that tribal people who have only been on the paleolithic diet are slimmer, stronger and healthier compared to those who aren't on the diet. These people do not suffer with cavities, dental problems, and have straight teeth. They also have perfect eyesight, rarely battle with arthritis, diabetes, obesity, heart disease, stroke, depression, cancer, and hypertension and schizophrenia disorders. There are approximately 84 tribes of hunter-gatherers left in this world who eat a Paleolithic diet. These people get daily adequate exercise which also helps them to stay healthy too. The tribal people have never evolved further like current civilization has done. The paleolithic diet is an advanced nutritional plan using wild plants and animals of different species. This diet has been around for over 2.5 million years however it ended 10,000 years ago when agriculture was developed. The Paleolithic diet theory introduced dieters with features of holistic and, comprehensive dietary combined together.

Why Go the Paleolithic Route?

The paleolithic diet should provide everything that the body needs to function properly. The primary dietary components are all covered, such as vitamins, phytosterols, proteins, fats, carbohydrates, and antioxidants. This diet is needed as it is programmed within our genes to eat these types of foods and discard foods that do not fit within the paleolithic diet.

Indigenous cultures that are around in this present day still eat the same diet of foods they have eaten for centuries have been considered primitive for not changing their diets. Instead these hunter-gatherers eat the foods that are in their area don't suffer what modern eaters suffer with today. Anthropologists has studied and compared these people with modernized people and they found that the results in association between diet and disease is completely clear that diseases such as diabetes, heart disease, cancer, arthritis and many other diseases were rarely found among the hunter gatherers.

Many dieters found that, after eating Paleo for three weeks:

- BMI dropped by about 0.8
- Average weight loss was around 5 pounds
- Blood pressure fell by an average of three mmHg
- Increase in antioxidants
- Healthier potassium-sodium balance
- Levels of plasminogen activator inhibitor (blood thickening agent) dropped by 72%.

Benefits of the Paleo Lifestyle

The top benefit of the paleolithic diet are eating foods that are naturally high in fiber. Fiber helps to reduce constipation, lower cholesterol, and lowers risks of diabetes and coronary heart disease. The paleolithic diet focuses on helping people lose weight with eating foods that were available during the Paleolithic era. These foods consist of meat, eggs, vegetables, roots, fish, mushrooms and berries. Our bodies are designed to handle foods loaded in high protein, and low carbohydrates however we are not genetically ready to handle low protein and high carb diets during these modern times. Eating a natural diet instead of a diet filled with processed foods, sugar-filled, and grain products.

The paleolithic diet offers the body a higher proportion of fat compared to the average Western diet. This higher proportion gives the body an additional health benefit of providing more energy and helps the body perform better. The fat found in modern diets is primarily unhealthy, consisting of a lot of trans fats. The quality of fat a body needs to consist of fat soluble nutrients including vitamins A, D, E, and K and the CoQ10 (coenzyme) can't be absorbed without the presence of fat. All of these vitamins are very important for the body and avoiding nutrient deficiencies.

Omega-3's provides many benefits for the body such as helping to increase brain size, and forming brain tissue. The omega-3 fatty acids are essential in supporting biochemical processes, creating membranes in cells which keep tissues healthy and maintaining the body's metabolism. It not only improves physical health but also improves mental health, build immune system, cardiovascular strength, and healthy digestion.

Paleo Food Types

Foods to eat

The paleolithic diets come into different types of restrictions depending on the dieter's preferences. The basic paleolithic diet consists of eating foods that are as close to nature or as natural as possible. These foods include:

- Meats – lean beef, chuck steak, lean veal, long broil, top sirloin, chicken, fish, pork, seafood, etc.
- Other Meat – venison, alligator, bison, reindeer, rabbit, pheasant, wild turkey, wild boar, goal, rattlesnake, emu, caribou, etc.
- Vegetables -
- Fruits
- Nuts & seeds
- Seed oils – olive, avocado, palm, coconut, almond, walnut, pecan, macadamia, hazelnut)
- Water
- Coffee and tea - drink the coffee black or with unsweetened almond milk

Foods to avoid

- Grains – barley, oats, rice, wheat, maize, rye, wild rice, millet, corn, etc.
- Grain-like Seeds – buckwheat, quinoa, amaranth
- Sugar – soft drinks, fruit drinks, candy, honey
- Legumes – all beans, lentils, miso, etc
- Dairy – butter, cheese, ice cream, milk, yogurt, creamer
- Any processed foods

Paleo Confusion

How to know if a food type adheres to the paleo plan.

There are many continuous ongoing debates on whether a certain food type adheres to the paleo plan as the diet focuses on what the first people ate before farming began. However, research is being done to find out if the first people ate potatoes. However, most speculate they did. The confusion comes from certain foods that can't really be classified as Paleo or not, like honey, oats or potato. The truth is, that the paleolithic diet plan isn't completely cut and dry. Saying that, most of the foods listed as paleo provide enough variety and satiety to continue with, without feeling like "cheating".

Paleo Food List

All of the following foods are paleo friendly to eat.

- Protein
- Eggs
- Fish
    - bass
    - cod
    - mackerel
    - grouper
    - halibut
    - herring
    - red snapper
    - salmon

- Lean Beef and lean cuts
    - Steaks – flank and chuck
      Lean hamburger beef
    - Veal
    - Sirloin

- Lean Lamb
    - lamb chops and loin

- Lean Poultry
    - Chicken, hen and turkey breast

- Other Meats
    - bison – ostrich
    - elk - squab
    - alligator - goat
    - bear - goose
    - kangaroo - caribou
    - pheasant - rattlesnake
    - rabbit –quail

- reindeer - emu
- turtle – wild turkey
- wild boar - venison

- Shellfish
  - crab - clams
  - abalone - crayfish
  - lobster – shrimp
  - scallops - oysters
  - mussels

- Fats
  - Brazil nuts - almonds
  - Avocado - coconut
  - cashews – flaxseed oil
  - coconut oil
  - chestnuts

- Cold pressed nuts and seeds
  - walnuts
  - pecans pumpkin seeds
  - pistachios
  - pine nuts
  - sunflower seeds
  - sesame seeds

- Vegetables
  - cauliflower - celery
  - artichoke - asparagus
  - beet greens
  - beets - bell pepper
  - broccoli
  - Kale - Brussels sprouts
  - cabbage – carrots - tomato
  - endive - green onion
  - Kohlrabi - watercress
  - collards - cucumber
  - lettuce - mushroom
  - mustard greens

- onions - parsley
- parsnip - peppers
- pumpkin - rutabaga
- radish - seaweed
- spinach - tomatillos
- Swiss chard – squash
- turnips and turnip greens

- Fruits
  - apple - apricot
  - banana - blackberry
  - boysenberry - papaya
  - cantaloupe - cassava melon
  - cherimoya - cherries
  - cranberry - figs
  - gooseberry - grapefruit
  - grapes - guava
  - honeydew -lychee
  - lemon - lime
  - kiwi –orange -mango
  - nectarine -
  - passion fruit -plums
  - peaches - pears
  - persimmon - pineapple
  - pomegranate - strawberry
  - raspberry – tangerine
  - star fruit - watermelon
  - tangerine
  - rhubarb

Sample Daily Meal Plan for Beginners

It can be difficult coming up with an original menu plan and easily eat something that is not Paleo related. The best option is to create a menu plan that will help you to make some good food choices and consistently stay on your Paleolithic diet. Create a meal plan that will last for a week or two so if possible purchase at least two weeks worth of food. Keep in mind that it's okay you can skip a meal whenever you want as the Paleolithic diet isn't about eating three meals a day. In this sample menu day plan there are **three** meals and a snack added providing you with enough options to work and play around with it.

Sample Menu Day Plan:

	Breakfast	Lunch	Dinner	Snack
Monday	Berries with coconut milk and mixed nuts	Broccoli and Pine Nut Soup	Meatballs with Crunchy Sweet Potato Chips	Pistachio Salsa
Tuesday	Scrambled Eggs with Mushroom	Cucumber Hot Dogs	Pumpkin and Chicken Curry	Grilled Tomatoes
Wednesday	Salmon and Zucchini Fritters	Roast Vegetables in Orange and Rosemary	Chicken with Macadamia Topping	Nut Butter Cucumber Sandwich
Thursday	Mushroom and Meat Omelet	Dory with Beetroot Salad	Lamb Chops	Tomato Salsa
Friday	Lemon Pancakes	Moroccan Lamb with Squash	Chicken and Egg Salad with Almond Sautéed Sauce	Cashew Nut Dip

Eating Paleo in Day to Day Life

Restaurants and Eating Out

Paleolithic dieters need to find paleo food friendly restaurants and eateries that cater specifically to their diet. There has been a slow trickle of restaurants available catering to natural and raw foods for health conscious people. Avoid leaving your Paleolithic diet up to chance as the failure rates are high when that is done. Instead look into planning ahead by preparing a list of Paleo-friendly restaurants near your home and work. However, keep in mind that your social life is completely different compared to your Paleo ancestors so there will be a trade off of some sort involved. So look into minimizing the damage and try to find more desirable options on the menu and then tighten up on your diet for the next several days. Your ancestors they didn't have temptations all around them to pull them off of their diet however they didn't consider the Paleolithic diet as a diet but as a means of survival.

While out in restaurants, tell the waiter you have a

gluten allergy and that includes any grains. Be serious about the topic and they will know to take it seriously and make sure that nothing has touched a non-paleo food or product. Ask for your meal to be cooked with olive oil.

Social Eating

When out with friends do let them know that you won't accept any bad foods. They should know about your diet beforehand so that it will not be a surprise. This is especially important if you dealing with an autoimmune disease or a digestive problem, or are trying to lose weight. Bringing some food of your own will also help to alleviate any issues that may arise. Allow your friends to taste the food you're eating and it will give you an added topic to discuss with your friends.

Food Preparation

Food meal planning helps with knowing what to prepare and eat. The sample meal planner in this book helps in providing ideas and deciding on the best options. Preparing your meals ahead of time instead of cooking daily is a timesaver.

Meal Frequency and Amounts

A person should in general eat when they are hungry, however eating at least 3-4 times a day is a good way to go. It all depends on what you feel fits your overall needs and schedule. The idea on the amount of food to consume meets closer to the FDA's RDI (Recommended Daily Intake) measurements. For protein, individuals on a 2000 calorie diet may need approximately 50% of protein.

Recipe Ideas

Breakfast

Mushroom and Pine Nuts Scrambled Eggs

Ingredients

3 eggs
2 teaspoons of finely chopped onions
2 tablespoons of finely chopped chives
1 cup of slice mushrooms
1 tbsp of oil
1 tablespoon of pine nuts
Salt and pepper

Instructions

Place the oil in the frying pan on medium heat and fry the onions for at least 3-4 minutes until they are browned lightly then remove the mushrooms from the pan.

In a bowl whisk the eggs then pour it into the frying pan

while constantly stirring the eggs.

Add the chives when the eggs are almost cooked, allow
it to cook for another minute or until the eggs are finally
cooked.

Add in salt and pepper for flavor, then turn off heat and
add in mushrooms, and pine nuts before serving.

Salmon and Zucchini Fritters

Ingredients

1 ½ cups of almond meal
2 eggs
100g of thinly sliced smoked salmon
1 tbsp chopped dill
2 roughly grated large zucchini with the liquid removed
Salt and pepper
1 tablespoon of oil

Instructions:

Combine the eggs and almond meal in a medium bowl,
whisking both together until it is smooth.

Stir in the smoked salmon, dill, salt and pepper, and zucchini.

Place the oil in the frying pan over medium heat.

Spoon in approximately 1 tablespoonful of the smoked salmon combination into the frying pan. Make sure to allow it enough room for it to spread.

Fry the mixture for about 2-3 minutes on each side until completely cooked with a golden brown look.

Drain the fritter on either some absorbent paper or a paper towel.

Repeat the same process and add oil to the pan between each batch in order for it to cook properly.

Serve with a delicious green salad such as an arugula green salad.

Lemon Pancakes

2 eggs
1 tbsp of apple sauce
2 tbsp of lemon juice
1/3 cups of almond butter
1 tbsp of coconut oil

Instructions:

Combine all of the ingredients except for the coconut oil into a bowl.

Heat the coconut oil in medium heat in a frying pan. Spoon the pancake mixture into the frying pan.

Fry the pancake for about 1 minute before flipping it over to the other side. Cook for 1 minute on the other side. Serve pancakes and enjoy.

Lunch Recipes

Dory Fillet with Beetroot Salad

Ingredients for the fish:

2 dory fillets
Lemon juice
Salt and pepper

Ingredients for salad:

½ small beetroot – diced finely
½ medium tomato –diced finely
1 cup finely chopped lettuce
5 chopped walnuts
Lemon juice

Instructions:

Preheat oven to 350⁰F degrees Fahrenheit.

Place the dory fillets in an oven tray and sprinkle it with salt, pepper and lemon juice.

Bake the fish in over for approximately 10-15 minutes.

For the salad, place all of the salad ingredients into a bowl combining them well and add in the lemon juice to taste. Serve the salad with fish and enjoy.

Cucumber Hot Dogs

Ingredients:

4 small sausages
4 small cucumbers
Tomato sauce (optional)

Instructions:

Preheat the grill medium/high heat.
Grill the sausages for about 6-8 minutes or until they are cooked thoroughly.

For the cucumber, cut the ends off the cucumbers and use a small knife or butter knife to remove the seeds by twisting the knife around in circles.

Place a hot sausage in the hollow part of the cucumber and serve with tomato sauce.

Dinner Recipes

Chicken Curry with Pumpkin

Ingredients

5 cups of diced pumpkin
Sliced 2 chicken breasts
2 tablespoons of olive oil
1 diced onion
2 finely chopped up garlic cloves
2 tablespoons of ground ginger
1 tablespoons of ground turmeric
2 tablespoons of ground coriander
2 tablespoons of ground cumin
Vegetable stock 1 ½ cups
1 small fresh heap of coriander, chopped
Add in a dash of salt.

Instructions

Put the diced onion and garlic into a pan, fry with the oil for at least 2-3 minutes on medium heat setting. Add in the sliced chicken and cook consistently stirring for about 10-11 minutes or until chicken has cooked thoroughly becoming white.

Add in the diced pumpkin, turmeric, ginger, cumin, and coriander. Stirring for at least 1 minute.

Add in the vegetable stock and allow it to simmer for approximately 15 minutes on low heat. Add in the chopped coriander, cover the pan and cook for about 2 minutes.

Add a dash of salt to taste.

Sides

Soups and Salads

Broccoli and Pine Nut Soup

Ingredients

1 diced onion
1 tablespoon of oil
3 cups of broccoli
3 cups of vegetable stock or chicken stock
¼ cup of pine nuts

Instructions:

Put the oil and diced onions in a large pan on medium heat until the onions are lightly browned.

Add in the stock and broccoli to the pan and let it simmer for approximately 10-15 minutes or until the broccoli has softened. Let the broccoli cool slightly.

Place the broccoli and stock into a food processor or use

an electric blender if you don't own a food processor to create a smoother texture.

Heat the soup and serve.

Roast Vegetables in Orange and Rosemary

(Serves 4-6)

2 cups of diced pumpkin
2 tbsp of olive oil
2 cups of diced sweet potato
1 cup of diced carrots
1 juiced orange
6 tbsp of fresh rosemary leaves
2 finely chopped garlic cloves
Salt and pepper

Instructions

Pre-heat a fan-forced oven to 400 degrees Fahrenheit.

Combine all of the ingredients together and place into

an oven proof dish

Bake in oven for 15 minutes. Remove from the oven and stir well to cover the vegetables in the orange liquid then return back to the oven for another 10-15 minutes or until the vegetables are tender.

Meats

Crunchy Sweet Potato Chips with Meatballs

Ingredients

Mince meat - 250g
Almond meal - 1/3 cup
Baby spinach – 3 cups
Tomato paste – approximately 25g
2 tablespoons of fresh sage
1 medium sweet potato
Olive oil
Salt to taste

Instructions

Preheat the oven to 350 degrees Fahrenheit.

Placing the spinach in a bowl, cover it with boiling water. Cook spinach for 2 minutes before draining out as much liquid as possible from the spinach. Chop the spinach.

Place the mince meat, chopped spinach, almond meal, dash of salt, sage, and tomato paste. Combine the entire ingredients well.

Heat the frying pan to handle deep frying and peel the sweet potato with a vegetable peeler into ribbons. Place a handful of the sweet potato ribbons into the frying pan for about 2 minutes. Allow them to brown slightly. Remove the cooked sweet potato ribbons and place on a plate with a paper towel on it to drain remaining oil.

Roll the mixture into 2.5cm size balls and place them on a baking tray lined with baking paper.

Bake in the oven for 10-15 minutes or until browned and cooked thoroughly.

On a plate place the meatballs with the sweet potato ribbons top of them.

Peppered Steak

Ingredients

4 - 100g rump steaks
Crushed peppercorns 4 tablespoons
1 beaten egg
1 tbsp oil

Instructions

Immerse the steak into the egg mixture, and then cover with crushed peppercorns.

Put the steak into pan or barbeque grill with some oil to grease. Fry on high setting for about 30 seconds on each side, then reduce down the heat and cook until steak is cooked tenderly.

Eat with boiled vegetables and/or crispy green salad.

Paprika Lamb

Ingredients

2- 400g cans diced tomatoes or 3 cups fresh tomatoes
2 tablespoons of olive oil
500g of lamb, diced
1 large onion, sliced thinly.
3 finely chopped garlic cloves
½ teaspoon caraway seeds
¼ cup of ground paprika

Instructions

With the oil in the pan add in the veal, set to medium heat and fry until browned. Save the pan juices to use as a sauce.

Remove veal from pan and add remaining oil along with garlic and onion. Put it on medium heating and cook veal for at least 4-5 minutes or until onions are soft. Add in the caraway seeds and paprika and stir for about 30 seconds.

Add in the veal and diced tomatoes to the pan, cover and leave to simmer for about an hour or until meat is tender and the sauce has thickened. If the sauce begins to dry then add in a little water to the mixture.

Moroccan Lamb with Squash

Ingredients

500g of lamb diced
1 tablespoon oil
Chicken or vegetable stock – 3 cups
1 tbsp ground cinnamon
3 cups of pumpkin diced
1 sliced onion
Cut into halves 6 yellow button squash
1 juiced lemon
1 tablespoon of honey
2/3 cups of prunes, pitted
Salt and pepper to taste

Instructions

In a pan heat oil, fry up the diced lamb until it has been cooked thoroughly.
Add in the chicken or vegetable stock and cinnamon.
Cover the pan and simmer for at least an hour.

Add in the squash, onion, pumpkin, honey and lemon juice, then cover again and simmer for at least a half hour, or until vegetables have been cooked. Add in salt, pepper, and prunes, and cook for about 5 minutes.

Allow it to cook before serving.

Poultry

Chicken with Macadamia Topping

Ingredients

2 teaspoons of olive oil
2 chicken breasts cut into 3 parts

For the Macadamia Topping:

1/3 cup of red onion diced
1 chopped finely garlic clove
1 teaspoon of the oil of your choice
Salt
½ cup of macadamia nuts
4 tablespoons of chives, chopped

Instructions

Put the pan on high setting, fry chicken with the oil. Cook the chicken for about 5-11 minutes or until the chicken is cooked thoroughly and browned. Cook both sides of the chicken.

For the macadamia topping, fry the onion, salt, garlic and oil separately until the nuts are soft and browned. Remove ingredients from the pan but leave the oil in it. Put the pan back on the heat and add in the macadamia nuts. Stir the nuts regularly until they are browned lightly. Use a blender to mix garlic and onion and nuts and pulse the blender until a crunchy texture has developed. Put the mixture into a bowl and combine in the chopped chives.

Sprinkle a sizeable amount of the macadamia combination over the chicken on a plate.

Serve the dish with steamed vegetables and a green salad.

Orange Chicken with Basil

2 tablespoons of olive oil
1 cup of orange juice, freshly squeezed (used oranges)
2 chicken breasts
Sea salt
Fresh basil 2/3 cup chopped roughly

Instructions

Pre-heat oven to 350⁰ degrees Fahrenheit.

Using 2 pieces of baking paper place the chicken breasts into them. Bash the chicken breasts with a meat hammer until they are at least 1cm thick. Use a meat hammer or the end of a rolling pin and bash chicken breasts until 1cm thick.

Place the chicken breasts into an oven dish along and add in the basil, olive oil, orange juice, and a good dash of sea salt. Using aluminum foil, cover the oven dish tightly. Bake in oven for about 30-40 minutes, or until it is cooked thoroughly.

Serve with a salad or steamed vegetables.

Avocado Sauce with Baked Chicken

Ingredients:

Largely chopped pumpkin at least 3 cups
1 tablespoon of olive oil
2 chicken breast fillets
½ of an avocado
1 tablespoon of finely chopped fresh basil
Salt and pepper
1 cup of fresh rocket leaves
1 tablespoon of lemon juice

Instructions:

Pre-heat oven to 350⁰ degrees Fahrenheit.

In an dish oven proof, put the pumpkin, salt and pepper, and olive oil. Bake for approximately 35-60 minutes or until completely cooked.

In medium heat, put the olive oil in a pan, fry chicken for about 4-8 minutes on each side or until cooked completely. Set the chicken aside for 5 minutes, then cutting across the grain, slice the chicken thinly.

In a blender or food processor, put the basil, lemon juice

and avocado, pulse until a smooth paste has formed.

Put the chicken over the pumpkin and add the rocket leaves and add the avocado sauce.

Bombay Chicken Skewers

Ingredients

6 wooden skewers (soaked in cold water for about 20-30 minutes)
2 diced chicken breasts
4 tablespoons oil
2 tablespoons sweet paprika
1 tablespoon ground cumin
1 tablespoon ground coriander
2 finely chopped cloves of garlic
1 tablespoon ground turmeric

Instructions

Pre-heat oven to 350°degrees Fahrenheit or pre-heat grill on high setting.
To make sauce heat oil and spices in a frying pan on medium heat for 2-3 minutes, or until fragrant.

Line an oven tray with baking paper and then thread chicken on skewers. Coat chicken well with sauce.

Bake in oven for approximately 30-40 minutes, or until chicken has completely cooked.

Cook chicken for 4-7 minutes on each side if using a grill.

Rosemary and Lemon Chicken Skewers

Ingredients:

6 wooden skewers (soaked in cold water for about 20-30 minutes)
2 diced chicken breasts
2 tablespoons rosemary, finely chopped
2 tablespoons olive oil
1 tsp grated lemon rind
1/3 cup of lemon juice
Salt for taste

Instructions

Pre-heat oven to 350°degrees Fahrenheit or pre-heat BBQ grill on high.
Place rosemary, lemon rind, olive oil, lemon juice and salt in a small bowl and combine together.

Thread chicken on skewers and put in a tray oven proof lined with baking paper, coat the chicken with lemon sauce and rosemary. Bake in the oven for about 30-40 minutes, or until chicken has thoroughly cooked.

Cook chicken for 4-6 minutes on each side if cooking on a grill.

Snacks

Pistachio Salsa

Ingredients:

1/3 cup of toasted pistachios
1 cup finely diced tomatoes
1 finely chopped large garlic clove
1/3 cup of roughly chopped fresh parsley
2 finely chopped mint leaves,
1 tbsp of lemon juice
Dash of round paprika

Instructions:

Combine all ingredients in a bowl and mix together well.

Tomato Salsa

Ingredients:

1 cup finely diced tomato
¼ cup of finely chopped red onion
1 ½ tbsp of ground paprika
½ tsp of Mexican chili powder
1 tsp of finely chopped tarragon or oregano
1 tbsp lemon juice
1 tsp vinegar (optional)

Instructions:

Combine all ingredients in a bowl and mix together well.

Cashew Nut Dip

Ingredients:

2/3 cup of unsalted cashews
1 tbsp of olive oil
3 tbsp lemon juice
Salt and pepper for flavor

Instructions:

Use a blender to combine all of the ingredients together until a smooth paste has formed.

For a crunchy texture then blend the ingredients for a shorter period of time.

Desserts

Blueberry Sorbet
Ingredients
2 cups blueberries
½ medium banana
1/3 cup of coconut milk
1½ tbsp honey
1 egg white, beaten until stiff peaks have formed

Instructions

Use a blender to blend together blueberries, banana, coconut milk and honey until well combined.

Fold blueberry mixture into the beaten egg white. Pour into an ice-cream container or a freezer proof container and freeze for approximately 6 hours or overnight until set.

To serve, cut into slices.

Stir in shredded coconut and then fold mixture into the beaten egg white.

Pour the mixture into an ice-cream container / freezer proof container and freeze for approximately 6 hours or overnight until set.

To serve, cut into slices and enjoy.

Mixed Berry Compote

Ingredients

2 tea bags herbal tea, such as chamomile, orange tea, jasmine
1 freshly squeezed orange
2 cups mixed berries

Instructions

Place tea bags and orange juice in a saucepan and simmer over low heat for 1 minute.

Add in the berries and allow it to simmer until berries are juicy and plump.

Take out the tea bags.

Cover and refrigerate for several hours prior to serving.

Paleolithic Cookbook Conclusion

The Paleolithic diet isn't a diet that is going to fade away but instead will continue to grow as more people gain knowledge about the full benefits of the diet. The fundamentals of the paleolithic diet provide dieters with the needed guidelines and principles to apply to our daily life and lifestyle. Our ancestors' diet may have varied as it depended on where they lived along with their environmental climates and other factors involved. Ancestors living around Canada would more likely eat fresh salmon, deer, berries and plants. Ancestors living in Africa would eat animals and plant roots. Aboriginals in Australia would live off the land eating plants, bugs, native nuts, honey and animals. Remember our ancestors ate well and were in good health and this same diet will provide the exact same benefits for us.

CPSIA information can be obtained
at www.ICGtesting.com
Printed in the USA
BVHW041230190122
626621BV00012B/1243

9 781631 877957